I'll Be Seeing You

A Wife's Journey With Her Husband's Alzheimer's

By Deane Johnson

Deane Johnson

This book is dedicated to:

David W. Moreledge M.D.—Joe's neurologist who has held our hand during this long journey.

To Dicque Barton Peterson—my cousin who has felt my pain along the way.

And to Jonathan Hal Reynolds, who helped to see this manuscript through to fruition and brought me a dozen red roses to celebrate.

Thank you all for encouraging me to finish this book.

Forward

Life is composed of a series of memories that we, as human beings, hope to cherish forever. Our first date, that first promotion, the big wedding day, or the birth of our children. When our brain is robbed of that ability to retain new memories due to a neurodegenerative process such as Alzheimer's disease, the patient's view of the world is considerably different than that of the caregiver's. The Alzheimer's victim is oblivious to his or her predicament, living each day like it's a new adventure. The caregiver and family bear the burden of dealing with a new and different individual, one who sadly regresses eventually to the level of a small child, being stripped of their own identity and God-given talents. There are currently over 5.3 million people in the United States living with Alzheimer's dementia. It is estimated that nearly 15 million family members and friends provide 24-hour care for these patients, impacting their own personal lives both emotionally and financially. The economic costs are staggering, rising from 183 billion dollars this year to more than one trillion by 2050.

However, I do have good news. We have made significant strides in the last 30 years in understanding the healthy human brain and how Alzheimer's disease affects it. We now know that certain pathological changes in the brain such as beta-amyloid, the main component of plaques, and the tau protein, the key component of neurofibrillary tangles, play vital roles in the interruption of vital cell transport and ultimate cell death. Other factors contributing to Alzheimer's brain pathology include cellular inflammation and insulin resistance, i.e., how brain cells use sugar and its substrates to produce energy. There are medications being developed that will target these abnormal cellular functions and hopefully offer disease modification rather than just mediocre symptomatic therapy. The two limiting factors that exist today in Alzheimer's research are lack of volunteers for clinical trials and inadequate federal funding. The secretary of Health and Human Services recently announced that an additional $50 million will be put toward Alzheimer's research over the next several months, and an additional $106 million will be given to caregiver support and education over the next year.

This book is written for anyone affected by this unrelenting, take-no-prisoners disease known as Alzheimer's dementia. The pages which follow are a true account of everyday life, full of real emotions, sometimes humorous situations, and gut wrenching reality. I applaud Deane for her candid account of her personal journey with this disease. Most importantly, I admire her for the wonderful caregiver she has been to Joe throughout this ordeal. I feel honored to be part of the story.

-David Morledge, M.D.

Writing does not eliminate my anxieties.

Writing helps me accept the changes that occur.

In the process of living and growing

And accepting life's ups and downs,

Writing helps me understand.

And understanding lessens my anxieties.

Deane Johnson
June 1988

"I'll be looking at the Moon, and I'll be seeing you . . ."

Introduction

When my husband, Joe, retired, we were looking forward to getting back to the adventurous life we had shared fifty years before as newly-weds. We had big dreams of traveling to far off places and sharing new exciting journeys. But then we found out Joe had Alzheimer's.

As we set sail into these uncharted waters, I searched and searched for information about the early onset of the disease. I found only clinical books, but nothing available on a personal level. It was then I decided to write something about the daily journey shared by the Alzheimer's patient and the caregiver. So in 2004, I began journaling daily to gauge Joe's progression down the path of Alzheimer's.

I have learned many things these past seven years. I have learned to be more patient and selfless, and that my love for Joe has only grown during this trying season. I've learned to find pleasure in simply being together, holding hands and exchanging a hug or a kiss. I've learned to live in the moment.

When our journey with Alzheimer's first began, I didn't know how to speak its language. But through the years, I have learned to speak Alzheimer's. And I hope my journal entries help you learn to speak it too.

-Deane Johnson

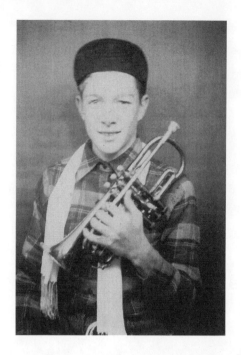

Joe, age 12, with his brother's Cornet.

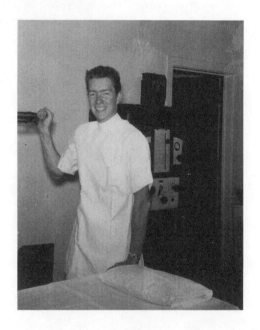

Joe at Providence Hospital as X-Ray Tech.

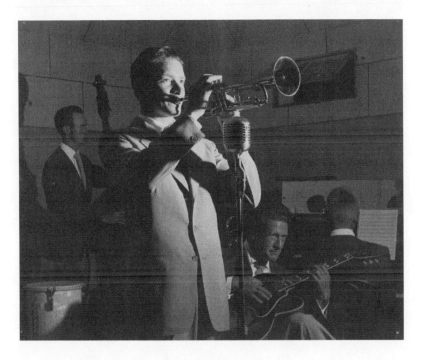

Joe Johnson Orchestra, April 1951. At Casa Blanca.

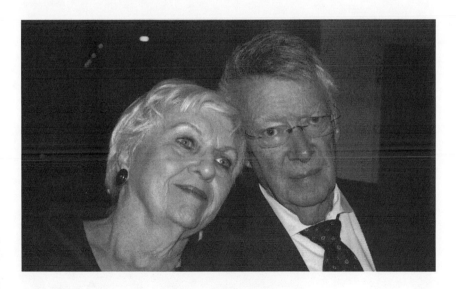

Joe and Deane at the last dance Joe ever played.

The Journal
(2003-2010)

January 1, 2003

Like a fly on the wall, I watch my husband meeting his days of retirement with apprehension. Each day lies ahead of him like an endless road to nowhere. Breakfast lifts his spirits momentarily, but once breakfast is finished and the paper is read, the long day spirals ahead of him once again.

I ask myself every day, What is plaguing Joe? Is he turning into the Absent-Minded Judge? Is he so bored with retirement that he has become lost? Is his problem dementia, aging, or just a severe case of daydreaming? Or is it something no one can label?

I have recently read about the early symptoms of Alzheimer's disease (AD). Out of 12 or more symptoms, only three apply to Joe. Personally, I rule out AD, but then I ask myself, *Am I in denial?*

This talented man retired on December 31, 2002. He was an icon of his community, having had success in all of his life's endeavors. He has been admired for his musical talent since the age of fourteen. Most musicians are speechless listening to Joe play jazz, or anything else for that matter. He was a knowledgeable x-ray technician, liked by doctors and nurses alike. He made lifelong friends in the Army, was a talented radio and TV newsman, a journalist, and a natural politician. For twenty-seven months he met the challenges of Law School while working a full time job as Justice of the Peace, booking and leading his band, and finding time to be a husband, father, and provider. He held the position as Justice of the Peace (JP) and was a full time practicing Attorney for twenty-four years. After nearly a quarter of a century as JP, Joe won his election for District Judge by a two to one margin, and presided in the 170th District Court for sixteen years. Joe has had more than his share of publicity and pictures in the *Waco Tribune Herald* and also on television. But in retirement, his days are empty compared to the life he has led.

"*Now what?*" he seems to constantly be asking.

I have tried to get him involved in different hobbies, but nothing interests him.

I am frightened thinking about our future.

The first worrisome trait both Joe and I noticed was that he had difficulty remembering names. We all do that at times, but his forgetfulness was something more extreme. He began asking me the same question several times within a matter of minutes. I rationalized that I had no right to expect him to remember where things were located around the house, because the house has been *my* office for over 50 years. He is retired, and thus, a newcomer to homebound existence. During the decades while he was working, our time together was in the evenings, on the weekends, and during our yearly vacation. Evenings were filled with laughter, TV, and a hot meal. Weekends were filled with church, golf, and TV. Our four weeks of vacation each year were always happy times full of fun, leisure, and relaxation.

But one morning, Joe woke up and the monotony of having nothing to do was a burden instead of a pleasure. He had to fill up the blank pages of the day which seemed much the same as the day before. My days had not changed, because I was still doing my work in and around the house, just as I had been doing for half a century. In the beginning, Joe enjoyed his leisure. He would sleep late, and sometimes so would I. We enjoyed sitting at the bar eating breakfast together, having several cups of coffee, and perusing the newspaper. We still do that, but Joe is sad now, and seems lost. He seems as if he is all alone in the world. I want to help him, but I don't know how. Since his retirement, we have taken trips to Vegas, spent six weeks in Europe, and enjoyed weekends in Dallas. As long as we are active, Joe seems content. But once all the motion ceases, he is lost once again.

January 2003

A brief summary of the past 9 months:

Excitement was in the air on the first day of Joe's retirement. Our plan was to pick up our lives where we left off over fifty years ago. Joe's career and our season as active parents had come to a close. Both jobs had been done well, and the future was now ours to relish and enjoy.

We slept late, enjoyed our morning time together, and looked forward to the rest of the day. During those first days, this was satisfying to Joe. But as one month ran into the next, Joe faced long days with nothing to do but sweep the patio, pick up trash in the yard, practice his horn, and watch golf and reruns of car races. There were no deadlines, no conferences, and no phone calls. Sometimes he sat in court as a visiting Judge, but that was not satisfying to him.

Spring rolled around and Joe sometimes played golf, but not on a regular schedule. He also played with local bands. He and I went to a few movies, and ate out several times a week as he tried to adjust to being home every day. From January 2003 until our Vegas trip in November, Joe traveled through a long dark tunnel. It was during this period when I first noticed Joe asking the same questions over and over. For example, he would forget where the flashlight was, even though he had just used it the day before. If he finally found the flashlight, he would again forget where he had found it. I noticed he left drawers and closet doors open, and would forget to give me phone messages. He forgot to go to Rotary, to haircut appointments, and he even forgot the names of people he had known for years. I have constantly asked myself if these are red flags. So what does it all mean?

November 2003

Joe had a thorough examination early in the month, and was diagnosed with the early onset of Alzheimer's disease. I was not convinced, but there have been times a red flag has gone up, and it has scared me. I don't like what I've read about AD. I have probably been keeping my head stuck in the sand, but who can blame me?

Dr. Paul Hurd asked the usual "memory questions." Joe did extremely well on the memory questions, and then Dr. Paul Hurd asked him to draw the face of a clock. Joe drew a round circle, thought for a moment, then drew all twelve numbers on the right side of the clock starting with one at the top and ending with twelve where six belongs. Jody looked at me, and I stared back at him. I took a deep breath, wondering what it all meant. I listened, and began looking for holes in the diagnosis. I made excuses, and refused to accept such a future. Can I be loving and caring and patient with this person I love so dearly? One might think it to be a foolish question. It is, and it isn't.

Dr. Hurd gave Joe samples of Aricept.

An appointment was made for November 21, 2003 for a complete examination, an MRI, and an EEG. It was then that the diagnosis was confirmed. Joe had 15% more atrophy in one portion of his brain than an average seventy-five year old man. The doctor then added 10mg of Namenda to the Aricept prescription.

It was also this month that we finally made our much-awaited trip to Las Vegas, and had a great time. Joe was alert, involved, and the trip felt much like all the other trips we've taken in the past. He had no trouble playing 21 or Craps.

When we checked into our hotel, Joe did not make a mental note of our room number. While I was unpacking, he decided to go down to the Casino. After I finished unpacking, I walked downstairs, and Joe was just standing in the long hall next to the Café. He didn't know our room number. My first thought was, *Is this for real?* I then decided he had been so anxious to go to the Casino that he had forgotten to pay attention to our room number. Am I making excuses? Am I still in denial?

Jan. 5, 2004

E-mail from Jody:

Mom, this book, Learning to Speak Alzheimer's *by Joanne Coste, is valuable information on daily questions. I continue to believe that the more knowledge we have, the more we will be able to help Dad, you, and the entire family. Love, Jody*

February 2004

The end of 2003 and the early months of 2004 have been unchanging. This month, we took another five-day trip to Vegas. I was convinced that having something to look forward to would be beneficial to Joe, as well as to me.

May, 2004

Joe and I are looking forward to our second visit to Paris, France. We had our second honeymoon in Paris in 1952. He was stationed in France and was working as an x-ray technician at the 28th General Hospital in La Rochelle. We lived in Fouras, France.

Now, fifty two-years later, we are looking forward to another honeymoon in Paris. I have been busy all spring planning this European trip. We departed Waco on May 17th, and had ten full adventurous days in France.

In this journal, I am only going to cover a few high spots. We did the usual tourist things. We enjoyed the sidewalk cafés, walking the left bank, going up on the Eiffel tower, taking a trip to Versailles, and visiting Giverny, Claude Monet's home and flower garden. Joe and I also have an audio recording of our trip that is funny.

The morning we went to the Louvre Museum, Joe was talking to several other guests while I was getting information about the metro. The name of our hotel was the Opera Cadet, and that just happened to be the name of the metro stop we were using. When it was time to get off at the Louvre, Joe and I were waiting for the door to open so we could get off. Joe said to me, "Get off, Deane," and I did . . . But the door closed before Joe could jump out. This was around ten in the morning. I didn't know where the metro would take Joe, or where he would finally get off. I didn't know if he even knew we were going to the Louvre, and I didn't know if he knew the name of our original metro stop—"Opera Cadet," near our hotel. Joe had my purse with passports, Euros, and identification. I had nothing but the ticket stub from the metro. I walked all around outside the museum looking for Joe. By 4p.m., I decided I wasn't going to find him. I had no money and didn't know how I was going to get back to the hotel. I finally figured out I could slip under the turnstile, walk across the bridge, and catch the metro back to our hotel.

What if Joe couldn't figure out how to get back to the hotel? I thought, growing more and more certain that Joe did have Alzheimer's.

A little while later, I was sitting at a window at the front of the hotel and saw a man with a black and gold Nike jacket coming down the sidewalk. It was Joe. I met him at the door, and we both cried. The scene was straight out of a movie—tears, kisses, and hugs.

Joe explained to me how he had found his way back to the hotel. He had gone to a metro station to buy a ticket, and had found an Opera Cadet card in his coat pocket. A couple from Germany who spoke English helped Joe get a ticket and told him where to get off. I'm sure they could tell from the look on his face that he was stressed and worried about me. This German couple that spoke English were our guardian angels.

On another day, we had planned a day trip to La Rochelle and Fouras. We traveled by train to La Rochelle. I had made arrangements to rent a car, but when we arrived there, the place was closed. We rented a car from another car rental, and wrote down instructions on how to get back to our hotel. We soon became lost.

After a while, we finally decided if we could get back to the train station, we could just turn the car back in and take a taxi from the station back to our hotel. Joe stopped at a pub, went inside, and, with hand motions, drew shapes of a train in the air. No one spoke English. The men in the pub stared with stunned faces, so Joe came back to the car. He said we would drive until we ran out of gas. As we were pulling out, a guy hopped on his motorcycle and waved for us to follow him. He took us straight to the train station. Another angel was watching over us. We returned the car, and set out to find a taxi.

With no car, we would have to get a driver to take us to Fouras. Only, I didn't have enough Euros to pay for a taxi. The hotel wouldn't exchange our money, but they told us the local casino would change our dollars into Euros. There was a catch. We had to get $500.00 changed to Euros and gamble half of it. I told Joe the Lord was sending us a message. Before we left Paris that morning, a zipper broke on one piece of luggage. I decided we would get an early train back to Paris and scrap this particular part of the trip. When we arrived at the train station back in Paris, the line for a taxi was long. A gentleman approached us and offered to take us to the hotel in his car. Upon arrival at our hotel the gentleman charged us a lot more than a usual taxi ride.

We continued the last leg of our trip on the Eurostar from Paris to London. We had ten days in London. We took many tours, and the last day we had High Tea at the Ritz. The piano player was playing one of my favorite songs, titled *"Again"*, as we were being seated. Joe called the sandwiches "conversation sandwiches." He said you take a bite, talk a little while, and then take another bite. The high tea was a wonderful way to end our trip.

Pneumonia joined Joe from London to Waco. I have often wondered what our family and friends think of me taking Joe with Alzheimer's to Europe. If I were a fly on the wall, I am sure I would hear an assortment of opinions.

August 5, 2004

During these past months, Joe and I have made many jokes about his memory. At first, I heard frustration in my voice whenever he asked me the same question three or four times. I hope I'm doing better now.

We have been home from Europe for nine weeks, and I've noticed the days are getting longer and harder for Joe. It is taking him a long time to get back to where he was before we left. I am beginning to wonder if he will ever be the same again. This man who has been busy all his life has lost his motivation and his passion. He knows he should be more active, but he has no incentive.

I have no answers.

August 10, 2004

I watched an Oprah show about AD. The film showed extreme cases, which, as of now, do not apply to Joe. I have no resources in which to search for early signs of AD. One day I suffer anxiety thinking that Joe has AD, and then two days later he seems back to normal. I ask, what is "normal?" Here is a man who has worked for 61 years, and is now retired, with no place to go and not much to do. Joe has said he feels worthless and disconnected. He sits as a visiting Judge when he is needed, but he doesn't enjoy it at all. He doesn't make any goals for himself, nor does he know what he really wants to do. He loves his music, and still practices daily. But at this time in life, we are both in limbo. For him, it is a matter of having too much empty time on his hands. For me, it is fear.

Fall 2004

Football is going to save us. Eric and J.J. Johnson, our grandsons, will be playing several high school games this fall, and their brother Blake Johnson is playing for SMU this season. We have already attended several of the games. When Joe is with others, he appears to be more involved. Then the next day rolls around, he looks up, and it is just the dogs, the same wife, and a day without anything to do. I wish I knew how to help him deal with this downward spiral. I am upbeat 99% of the time, but I think that annoys Joe at times. Some days I feel like I'm married to Luna, my mother who always had the blues.

P.S. The day we went to see Dr. Hurd was a good day. Joe's memory test improved.

November 2004

The Burlesons joined us on our trip to Las Vegas earlier this month. Joe played poker the day we arrived, and continued to play constantly over the next five days. On the night we all went to Delmonico's, Ed asked me (instead of Joe) if he should put the charges on his own credit card and we could settle up later. I thought that, by Ed and me keeping up with the charges, it would be easier on Joe. That proved to be a big mistake. Joe accused me of having a thing going on with Ed.

Joe and I had three days by ourselves after the Burlesons left on Thursday morning, and he was my shadow until we left. He didn't play any more poker, yet blamed me for it, saying it was because I wanted him to be by my side. His disposition mellowed out upon our return home.

Not long after, we took a trip to New York with a large group from the bank. Joe was dreading it. The Burlesons were there with us, and the four of us attended the theater to see *42nd Street*, the musical. During dinner on Monday night, Ed spoke to me about the check, and he and I decided we would settle up later. Joe was so angry. He, the head of our family, had been having trouble with numbers and receipts because of his Alzheimer's. I thought I was helping him by settling up with Ed, but looking back, I was unintentionally demeaning Joe.

The week before Christmas, I was walking on eggshells, and couldn't explain why. On Christmas Day, Jody and his family, and Barry and his family drove down to Waco. Joe enjoyed the conversations, the reminiscing, and the laughter. I thought everything was fine.

The Cowboy game came on at 3p.m., and I knew Joe had been looking forward to it. But before half time, the dogs began looking out the window toward the backyard. Joe was outside raking leaves.

A Dream

I had a dream recently that I was in my Aunt's house and couldn't find a way out. I knew where the doors were, but I couldn't get out. Several months later, I had a dream that was along the same premise. I was lost, but couldn't find my way.

My interpretation: I am in the house with Joe every day, and I don't know how to fix what's broken. We are trapped in this journey together with no map, and no directions.

February 2005

Some days, I am not certain that Joe has been diagnosed correctly. Then there are days I am completely lost, unsure of myself and not knowing what will happen next.

Examples:

1) Joe is the one who puts up the Cokes once I get back from the grocery store, yet every day he asks, "Do we have Cokes?"

2) His underwear have been in the same drawer for thirty-eight years, and he has to ask where his underwear are. He puts on slacks, but can't remember what closet they were hanging in when he goes back to hang them up at the end of the day.

3) The license plates on the Lincoln expired. We had not received a notice to get new license plates, only a letter asking if we wanted new plates. Joe said he didn't want to go to the Court House, so he sat in

the car, and I went in. Joe felt inadequate in the situation, because the things he has taken care of for years were difficult for him to handle. That night at dinner, he thanked me for taking care of everything, and apologized for putting the job on me. I told him that it was time for me to learn how to do the things, because he has taken care of for 53 years.

4) If we are watching a TV show with several plots, he will ask me if I am able to follow the story line. I notice that he will nap if the show is too involved. After watching a show, I have learned not to ask him anything about the plot or characters. He will tell me he wasn't paying attention.

5) Joe will talk to someone on the phone, and if I ask what they said, he doesn't remember. I have learned not to press the point. He also forgets to tell me if someone called for me.

6) I take care of our taxes and investments. It is too confusing for Joe, though he is with me when we meet with our accountant or banker. I want to include him in all decisions that we may need to make.

I could very easily get depressed reading the above examples, but I choose to see our lives as a gift. Joe is an easygoing, loving, and thoughtful man. He may not remember to surprise me or remember to buy "special occasion" gifts anymore, but he is all he can be in these waning years. I am fortunate, and as long as we can function we are going to travel, go to movies, and he will continue to play his trumpet. Our days will be filled with love, understanding, and appreciation for one another.

March 16, 2005

We went to dinner tonight for Dena's Birthday. Mindy talked to Joe on the phone and told him where we would meet. Joe told her that I would know where to go. During dinner, Jim asked Dena a question about a contract with the builder she was using. At that point, Joe turned his back to them and looked at me. I knew exactly what he was feeling. He had recently told Mindy that he felt out of the loop, and that no one came to him for advice any more. I tried to involve him by saying something like, "Joe, I bet you have heard these same kind of problems in your Court Room?" I was thinking maybe Jim or the girls would ask his advice. It never happened. This is why he feels out of the loop. I know it was unintentional, but I wish he would be included in any conversation about law or music. He is familiar with these subjects and has years of experience.

April 2005

The other night in bed I was reminiscing about eating at a very fancy restaurant at the Venetian Hotel in Las Vegas. Joe wanted to know exactly where the hotel was and where the restaurant was located in the hotel. He remembered the name of the restaurant, Del Monaco's, but did not remember eating there. We laid there watching TV, and Joe began to tell me about a particular guy at Del Monaco's dressed casual and wearing his cowboy hat while having dinner. This tells me that if he really thinks hard, he can recall things.

Recently, Joe asked the names of Dena's children. I told him to think of A, B, C, and D. He remembered Beau and Drake, but not Austin or Colby.

He can do many things without being reminded: Rotary, taking his pills morning and night, and doctor appointments. He is always clean, fresh shaven, and dresses very nice. On many days, he helps cook, clean, and even makes up the bed.

He practices his trumpet daily, and has an incredible musical memory. He can play and sing the intros, chorus, and bridge of any tune, though he may forget some of the lyrics. If he does forget, you wouldn't know it. He makes up lyrics as good as the original. Is it Alzheimer's, aging, or something else entirely?

May 2005

Our visit to Dr. Hurd this month was positive. Joe made the highest grade yet on his memory test.

I wrote a letter to each of the children about the visit. The letter follows:

May 23, 2005

Dear Jody, Barry, Mindy and Dena,

I started to say this would be a brief update about our visit with Dr. Hurd, but I don't think I have ever been brief.

On Friday, April 29, 2005, we dropped by Barry's office, and the three of us had lunch before our 2p.m. appointment. I had mentioned to Barry and also to Jody that I was uncomfortable talking about Joe when Dr. Hurd would ask me about my observations. As we were escorted to the room, Barry spoke to the nurse, relaying to her my apprehension. The nurse asked me to go to the front desk. She told me what Barry had told her, and I waited to have a private conversation with Dr. Hurd. I sat down in his office and froze. I did mention that I had my doubts about the diagnosis of AD, and that thought Joe had dementia. Dr. Hurd quickly told me that the test had ruled out dementia, and he was sure the AD diagnosis was on the money. He made a copy from a medical meeting explaining the difference. I told him we were planning several trips, and he encouraged me to keep Joe busy and on the go at this time. These activities are good for him. Then the doctor reminded me that this disease is fatal, and in time his personality may change. I was thinking, "How can that happen?" My husband, your father—talented, full of fun and a great sense of humor—will always have the same traits he has always had. I told Dr. Hurd that I did not want to think about such things for now. He then asked me if Joe is aware of this diagnosis. I told him that Joe never talks about it. The doctor began to fold the article for me to put in my purse so Joe wouldn't see the words, "Alzheimer's disease." I looked into the doctor's eyes and said, "I can handle this." I could not think clearly enough to ask any more questions. Fear silenced me.

Dr. Hurd joined Joe and Barry in the examining room. As soon as I stopped my overflow of tears, I joined them. Dr. Hurd was asking Joe about medications he takes. As soon as I walked in, Joe turned to me so I could answer the questions. Dr. Hurd gave Joe another memory test and was quite surprised that he had a higher grade on this test than all the previous ones. Joe drew another clock with all the numbers in their proper place. It is obvious that the medication is working. The only test question he had a little problem with was starting with 100 and subtracting by seven.

On the way to Dallas, Joe had asked me to question him about current events and dates. I was pleased the way he answered questions. In the doctor's office, he remembered not only the questions I had asked but was quick to answer different questions Dr. Hurd had asked.

We had a nice visit and left Dallas before 6p.m. Joe drove us, and we were home before 9p.m. On the way home, we talked about the good report he had received on his memory test. He never asked why I left the room while he was waiting to see Dr. Hurd.

Our days go quite well until our visits to Dr. Hurd. Joe's reaction to the visits is a tiredness he can't quite shake. Like me, I'm not sure Joe has come face to face with reality. Joe never talks about the rhyme or reason of the visits to Dr. Hurd. He simply goes, takes the tests, and leaves.

I found a Peanuts comic in the paper which I identify with. In the comic, it is pitch dark, and Snoopy is lying on top of the dog house. Snoopy is thinking; "What's that? I thought I heard a noise. These nights kill me. Everything seems so hopeless at night. What am I doing here? What's the purpose of it all?"

Snoopy worries about what might happen to him and what his master would do if he got sick or hit by a car.

Snoopy's last thought is, "People think dogs have no worries, and we don't as long as the sun is up." What a comfort to know Snoopy also dreads nighttime!

Joe and I are settled into our nightly rituals. He is always asleep within thirty minutes. I can't drop off to sleep that quickly. I find nighttime to be the darkest. My eyes well up with tears, but I know I can't cry because any movement or noise out of the ordinary wakes Joe. If I get up to go to the bathroom, blow my nose, or twist and turn, he asks if I'm okay. Joe pats me, and puts his hand on my back several times each night to make sure I'm breathing. I can't cry at night, because I don't want him to know that Fear crawls into bed beside me. And I can't cry in the daytime. Seeing my red eyes would alarm him, and I don't want him to know that I am worried about anything.

My goal is to discipline myself, to enjoy the moment, keep my mind in the present, and face tomorrow when tomorrow arrives. If I concern myself too much with what the future holds, I would miss the present times we have together. Each morning, throughout the day, and in the dark of the night, I ask for guidance, patience, and a hand to hold as we travel together on this journey. Am I facing my fears while enjoying each day as it unfolds? I hope I am. Tears are always just beneath the surface, and it is hard to avoid the fear that seems to shadow me. I fight it daily.

One is never too old to change, improve, and learn. I find myself on a difficult path, one I never expected to travel. On this journey, I must learn to be more patient—a quality I never had a good handle on, but one that I need to acquire. I am disciplining myself to answer the same question from Joe several times and not roll my eyes or give an audible sigh. I am in the driver's seat more than usual. I always thought it was where I belonged, but I find it to be lonely. Lonely or not, I will find my way. I am blessed to have my soul mate, Joe, and our four wonderful children on this journey with me.

I want to emphasize the importance of making your families your first priority. It is important to be active and involved with your mate and children. Every day is a building block day in the lives of your families. Call when you have a minute, and always make sure you visit with your dad. He would love talking with your mates and children too. Visit when you can. He enjoys seeing you anytime, with your families or alone.

You may have some questions you would like to ask him, or maybe just listen to a story you've heard before. There are so many things I wish I had asked my mother, Aunt Lela, and Joe's mother before they passed on. When I asked my mother how she had met my dad, she could not remember, but she was in her 80's before I ever asked. I don't know how mother Johnson met Roy B. I wish I had thought to ask. She did tell me they rode a streetcar to their apartment, and strawberries and cream were in the icebox waiting for them after their wedding ceremony. Now is the time to make a history connection with Joe. I don't think he will change much to the degree I read about in books about Alzheimer's. I hope I'm right. I will face tomorrow when tomorrow comes.

Joe and I are now past our autumn years. We are in our winter years. As we age, none of us think about facing anything more than cataracts, high cholesterol, maybe a minor problem with hearing or seeing, high blood pressure, brittle bones, glaucoma, and other problems that are part of aging. There is medication for these problems. But sometimes a shocking revelation comes from left field. This Horse named "Alzheimer's" is about to throw us to the ground.

I always envisioned us as aging, but remaining very active. I imagined us driving around the U.S., traveling to other parts of the world that interest us, strolling down the Champs Elysees, walking the left bank in Paris, watching grandchildren grow up, marry, and present us with great-grandchildren, and watching each of you become grandparents. We will continue to be active and travel for now. I am thinking that not much will change for eight to ten years, and if it does, we have made many memories to comfort us.

I was reading a devotional from the "Upper Room." I read the piece titled "Face the Fear." This family was vacationing at the beach. Their daughter, Sara, was afraid of the waves, but she finally ventured into the water and her parents could see her lips moving as she braced herself for each wave. When asked what she was saying, Sara said, "I just looked at the waves and kept saying, "Face the Fear," over and over again.

God did not give us a spirit of timidity, but a spirit of power, of love, and self-discipline.

From 2 Timothy 1:7.

I will not travel this road alone knowing I have God by my side, as well as our dedicated and loving sons, daughters, and friends. Fear is not welcome. I am comforted, knowing I have extra hands to help me if I stumble, and as time goes on I am sure I will take a few tumbles.

My, how I love you all.

Lovingly,
Mother

May 2005

Mother's Day came. The kids gave me a gift certificate. Mindy said she had asked Joe if he wanted to be included in the gift, and he said "no." That answer did not hurt my feelings. In church, Joe admires my jewelry and shows great pride in having given it to me, but the process of buying the gift grieves him. Do I wish he would plan something for me? Of course, but that is not going to happen. How could I expect him to remember special occasions when he doesn't remember current events, grandchildren's names, or what closet his suits are in?

As I sit here writing this journal, Joe is playing the trumpet, and his music brings me back to a special moment in time. He is playing "Stardust", and throughout the entire song tears blur my eyes. I now realize my daily gift is the music that floats from the bedroom as he plays. How could a gift wrapped in paper and ribbon top "Stardust?" I am a lucky gal.

We are planning another trip to Vegas in June. I also have tickets for another trip to Europe in September. Sometimes Joe doesn't seem interested in Europe anymore, but I know activity is good for him. When a lot of families hear the diagnosis, life comes to a halt for them. But I try to stay upbeat and to tell Joe how much I look forward to our trips. He follows along, because he doesn't want to disappoint me. Dr. Hurd's nurse thinks keeping Joe active will pay off just as it did on his recent memory test.

June 7, 2005—Tuesday

I sometimes ask Joe to feed the birds. I have two feeders. One is long and round and is filled with seed. Another feeder is a square cage that holds seed from a square package. Today, Joe took the square package of seed that fits in the square cage, and he was gone a long time. When he came back inside, he was hot and aggravated and said, "I can't get the seed in the bird feeder." I thought it was because he couldn't find the clip that opens the side of the cage, but that's not what he had done. He had tried to get a twelve inch square of solid bird seed into the six inch round hole of the feeder that holds loose seed. He was not amused, but I did laugh silently just visualizing him trying to put a twelve-inch solid square of bird seed into a round feeder with the opening about the size of a quart jar. Is this the mind of a 76-year old, or is it AD?

June 11, 2005—Saturday

Our trip to Vegas was fun this past week. Joe is himself when he is exposed to changes of scenery. He loves the electric vibration he gets when he gets caught up in the shows and all the activities in Vegas. We enjoy sitting outside at the sidewalk coffee shop just watching the people and planning our next move. We stay up late and sleep in every morning.

When it comes to organizing our lives, I am in charge whether I want the job or not. I accept the job of taking the lead, but I have to be honest—at times I find it overwhelming. I am responsible for making plans, buying tickets, making reservations, choosing where we eat, ordering medicine in advance, and all our other activities. I am the one who keeps tabs on all investments and banking. I never thought I was capable of doing all these jobs, but I am doing it. The one trait I have developed, and am still working hard at, is patience. Joe was naming my talents tonight, and twice he said, "My confidant." That told me that he doesn't want his problem discussed, and it is his way of saying, "You promised."

June 22, 2005—Wednesday

When Joe woke up this morning, I could tell it was going to be a hard day for him and for me. He sat with a sad face while eating his breakfast. Then he sat out in the garage by himself. I often try to help him find joy in his existence, and suggest things he could do to enjoy the day, but it usually falls on closed ears.

June 24, 2005—Friday

I had Joe make a list of three things he should do: go to the bank, run by the cleaners, and get the car washed. He decided to go to the bank at 3:30p.m. to deposit the traveler's checks we had purchased before we went to Europe. When he left, I asked if he had filled out his deposit slip, and he said he would do it at the bank. When he returned, I asked if he had deposited the traveler's checks, and he didn't know. His excuse for being unsure was that the bank was closing and he had to hurry. I asked if he had the deposit slip, and he began looking in his pockets. I told him he probably put it in his checkbook, and sure enough, that's where it was. How do I help Joe keep up with money and at the same time give him his independence and privacy? I don't think I know how to accomplish that. Maybe over time I will figure it out.

June 25, 2005—Saturday

This morning, Joe and I were having breakfast, reading the paper, and talking about our September trip to Europe. Joe suddenly frowned, and I assured him that our time in Paris was going to be more fun this year than it had been last year. He said he did not remember going to Europe last year. That shocked me. Finally, after we listened to the tape recordings we had made, he said he remembered.

July 2, 2005—Saturday

Joe drove himself to Burger King and he ordered a hamburger instead of a Whopper. The burger that he ordered only had meat and bread. He was upset, and made some comment about feeling out of touch with the world.

Later, I noticed that he had not taken his pills the night before (it is so important he doesn't miss his medicine). I had to approach this with gentleness, because a few nights before when he stepped out of the shower, I had reminded him to take his medicine. His reply had been, "You don't have to remind me. I am going to take the pills."

I am learning every day to be gentle. I am not perfect at this.

July 7, 2005—Thursday

Joe had a golf game this morning. Before he left, I reminded him that I would not be home when he returned. When I came back home later, he was standing in the kitchen next to some fast food napkins, and said to me, "I called to see if you wanted a burger. In fact, I called you *three* times. Of course, you're never home."

I said, "Joe, I was at the beauty shop."

He said, "How am I supposed to know your schedule?"

I then defended myself by saying, "I told you before you left to play golf that I would not be home when you finished." This comment was hurtful to Joe. After I said that, I suggested we both keep our thoughts to ourselves before one of us goes too far. I need to keep in mind that he does not remember these kinds of details. Every day I get a small glimpse into his world. With the presence of the Spirit in my life, I know I can meet these daily hurdles.

July 22, 2005—Friday

While Joe was shaving, I was bemoaning the fact that I have to go to the grocery store and my knees always hurt more after the trip. He always becomes a bit arrogant when I complain about anything that I have to do, and he is quick to remind me that he worked hard for forty years and we are still reaping the monetary rewards. My perception of that statement has always been that he doesn't give me any credit for my work at home with the kids all those years. Will I ever learn that defending myself brings out the rage in Joe? He grabbed me by the shoulder and was ready not just to hit me but also to walk out of the house. I sat very still, looked him square in the eyes, and firmly told him, "Don't go there." I went to the store, madder than h____. When I returned home, he was waiting at the gate to help unload the groceries.

August 5, 2005—Friday

Our grandsons, Austin, Beau, and Colby spent the night with us. Joe enjoyed his time with the boys.

August 8, 2005—Monday

I warned Joe last week not to trim the shrubs. But last Friday, he met me in the driveway when I pulled up, beaming with pride because he had finally finished trimming the last two shrubs. Now my Abellia and Bridal Wreath are squares. I am going to have to put warning signs or tags on each bush, reminding Joe not to trim them. Who am I kidding? That would never work.

August 12, 2005—Friday

Joe played a reunion concert with his band this evening, and it was a sellout. At the end of the night, he sang several songs. The words to "My Desire" will make your toes curl up.

> *"To spend one night with you in our old rendezvous*
> *And reminisce with you that's my desire."*

I know Joe is past reminiscing. Our current conversations are of the moment, and that is okay. Joe knows who I am most of the time, and I will not destroy each and every moment by crying over spilled milk.

Aug. 13, 2005—Saturday

We had brunch at a friend's house today. Lenny, a longtime friend of ours, approached me to inquire about Joe. I froze. I promised Joe I would not discuss his memory with anyone. I don't ever want to do anything to break Joe's trust in me, yet at the same time I know I need to confide in a friend. That is why I called Lenny tonight after Joe went to bed. Lenny, who has a PHD in psychology, said he had noticed a difference in Joe.

August 14, 2005—Sunday

Before we fell asleep tonight, Joe said, "Tomorrow is Monday and a long week lies ahead."

I replied, "It is a week to look forward to."

August 15, 2005—Monday

Joe sat out in the garage most of the morning, hot and steamy as it was, just staring into space. After we lifted weights, he seemed to perk up a little.

August 27, 2005—Saturday

Joe is content, but is having more trouble with his short-term memory. Is he slipping, or am I aware of every little thing? Luckily, Joe did show interest in reading about our upcoming trip to Europe.

September 2005

Our flight to Italy was somewhat enjoyable. I am so impressed with Joe when we are on a trip. I feel like I have the normal Joe back. Our tour of Italy went smoothly. We saw Rome, took a side trip to Pompeii, two days in Florence, two days in Venice, and on to Milan. Every day was busy and enjoyable, but Joe did not warm up to the others on the tour. He doesn't mind me being friendly, but he is standoffish. He finally warmed up toward the end of the trip.

Two couples picked up on Joe's memory problem. They were watching out for him, and several of the young girls took us under their wing. People we have never seen and will probably never see again were thoughtful and helpful. While I was napping on the bus one day, the tour director passed around a sheet of paper to get our addresses, phone numbers, and e-mail addresses to make copies for us to exchange. On the way to Milan, the tour director handed back the paper to all of us. Joe had put our address on Irving Lee, a street we lived on 39 years ago. He was horrified when he realized what he had done. And he was embarrassed.

Later that day, we had a late lunch in the hotel bar in Milan, and Joe began to cry. He said he didn't want to continue living if he was heading down such a road. I brushed it off as a mistake anyone would make. I made a reference to all the "bedroom activity" we enjoyed while living on Irving Lee, and told him that must have been what he had been thinking about when he wrote down that address.

We have tape recordings of our two week trip, a poem about Italy, and letters to grandkids about this trip. Maybe someday I will write details about both our 2004 and 2005 trips.

November 27, 2005—Sunday

A Birthday Greeting to Joe:

On November 27, 1951 we celebrated your 23rd Birthday and our one month Anniversary. I had $800.00 left over from my 21st Birthday gift of $1,000.00. I bought you three plaid shirts. For our Anniversary gift, I bought us a set of tea and juice glasses and a pitcher with your initials "JJ" embossed on the set. You told me your favorite cake was Angel food, so I beat twelve egg whites to perfection and baked you a birthday cake.

When I cut you a slice of cake, you looked at the cake, then up at me, and said, "I didn't mean Angel Food cake. I think my favorite is called Devil's Food Cake."

Now 54 years later.

Tonight when you reach for my hand while watching TV, I see you wearing the many hats you have worn through the years. I have a mental picture of you on the bandstand at Casa in 1950, of you in France wearing your hospital whites with that hat cocked to the side, of you rocking all our babies, and of you coming in the back door after a hard day at the Rock (Court House). In my mind, you will always be 23, in the way you express your love to me, show the softness of a young father, and the same sex appeal you have had since I first saw you in 1950.

Happy Birthday to my gift of a lifetime, my Joe.

Love,
Deane

December 29, 2005—Thursday

E mail to Jody, Barry, Mindy and Dena:

Today, I am taking down our Christmas tree, wondering what our lives will be like next Christmas when I put the tree back up. Lily, our Schnauzer is sick, and she probably won't be around next Christmas. Barry is in the belly of a divorce. Joe told Kenny that every time he looks at me, I am crying. I thought I was hiding my tears.

The road I am traveling is a daily exercise of self-discipline, not allowing myself to imagine what the next turn has in store for us, and demanding myself to relish each moment. Joe is a great guy. I am a lucky woman to be his wife, your mother, and "Gaga" (nickname) to this family. We may find ourselves in a valley right now, but there are still more mountain tops to cherish along this road called Life.

Love,
Mom

January 17, 2006—Tuesday

E-mail from Jody:

Mom, sorry it took so long for me to reply. I spoke to Dr. Hurd and to Audett Rackley at the Center for Brain health at the University of Texas in Dallas. At this time, there is not another drug for Alzheimer's although there is constant research going on. Audett said the most important thing that can be done for any level of dementia is to keep the patient active and stimulated. You are doing a great job in this regard. I talked to dad today and had a great discussion with him. I will see you soon.

Love,
Joe

Feb. 14, 2006—Saturday

E-mail to Jody:

Dear Jody,

I am thinking about a trip to Switzerland in 2007. I must keep Joe busy. On our trips, I make all the reservations and plans, and I keep Joe as close to me as I would a toddler. The time will come when long trips are no longer plausible, but, for now, it's good for both of us to travel.

May 11, 2006—Thursday

Today, Jody told me his wife had filed divorce papers in March. He wanted me to tell Joe. But when Barry brought Joe home, Joe kept saying, "Jody never said a word about his divorce."

I think Jody was fearful of breaking down and not knowing how it would affect Joe. I wish the boys would discuss their problems with Joe. I think it would be good for Joe to be in the loop even if he forgets it all by the next day. It would give him a chance to give some advice.

June 30, 2006—Friday

Joe is slipping a little faster than I had hoped. I think what I miss most is that the conversations we have today will be forgotten by tomorrow. If I remind him, sometimes he remembers.

There is one aspect of this disease that I view as a gift: the close relationship that has grown between us. I doubt we would be this close under normal circumstances. Our children tell me they see it too. I thank God for the chance to show by example. Ours is a love to be envied.

July 3, 2006—Monday

E-mail to Lenny:

Dear Lenny,

I hope you don't think I am spending my days grieving. I am facing this with a positive attitude. I am constantly aware that today is the best that this disease will be. This bump in the road has given me a chance to mature as a person.

This disease changes the person a little every day. One thing I have to work on daily is patience and self-discipline—i.e., always using a calm, loving voice when Joe asks me question after question.

Joe is still the man I fell in love with fifty years ago. He is funny, always mannerly, and is a perfect mate even with Alzheimer's. I tell our children I look at this disease as a sort of gift. Our relationship has grown to new heights. I think Joe and I are setting an example of a happy marriage through this journey. Robert Browning said it best:

"Grow old along with me. The best is yet to be.
The last of life for which the first was made."

I say, "Amen."

July 5, 2006—Wednesday

Rotary always meets on Monday, but for some reason Joe has told me several times today he is going to Rotary. I tell him this is Wednesday, not Monday. He says okay, then in five or ten minutes he tells me again that he is going to Rotary.

This morning, after taking his pills, he went back to the cabinet to get more pills. Joe completely forgot he had taken them. I am going to hide his pills and start giving them to him myself.

This disease is a long goodbye. I am thankful for every minute of every day that Joe and I spend together. I pray for my voice to be loving and caring each time I speak.

July 10, 2006—Monday

E-mail to Kathy:

Kathy,
*   Joe is sliding more than I thought he would. I worry about him driving. He doesn't remember our grandchildren's names or who their parents are. We are planning another trip to Vegas in September. I want to keep him busy and make sure he has something to look forward to. I'm trying to make the most of every day.*
*   Kathy, thanks for your "hand." It is an amazing comfort we human beings receive when holding a hand—e.g., a baby's hand when those little fingers grab our fingers, holding hands with our first love, and holding our mate's hand in the middle of the night. Your friendly hand typing a "Thinking of You" message to me is a powerful gesture. Thanks for holding my hand.*

God Bless,
Deane

July 16, 2006—Sunday

Joe forgets when he poops. He will tell me he hasn't been to the bathroom in days. I try to keep up with his visits to the bathroom, but he is so private he doesn't want to tell me.

August 5, 2006—Saturday

Joe may forget questions he has asked only a few minutes before, but he has no trouble remembering tunes, lyrics, and how to play the trumpet. It is amazing to watch this genius with Alzheimer's play and sing without hesitation. We are both excited about the band reunion tonight.

On a spiritual note, I have not been angry with God about Joe's Alzheimer's. I have never asked "Why Us?" But now I find myself angry with Joe. I clam up, not wanting to talk to him, and irritated even when he says things like, "You're my girlfriend, you belong to me, and you're my lover." I ask myself, "Why does this irate me?" Yesterday I sat in front of this keyboard and vented my anger loudly. Joe was outside. After my typing session, I felt calmer, but how long will the calm last? I know my job is to stay steady in the boat, loving Joe and learning to find joy in every day. I know that I control the level of contentment we both need. I know Joe can't help his loss of memory, and none of this is purposely done. But sometimes the angel on my shoulder is sleeping, and the devil goes to work on the tone of voice I use. The devil steals away my patience. I am responsible for all of Joe's maintenance like showering, giving him his medication at the right time, his three meals a day, and keeping up with his visits to the potty. I try to be as diplomatic as I can be in pointing out the dangers when he drives. When I am on my soap box with my gentle voice, he begins to whistle or hum. We are on a trip with no maps, although so far I've managed to find the way.

August 26, 2006—Saturday

Joe recorded his new album all day today. The day went by without a single bobble. I enjoyed every minute of it.

August 29, 2006—Tuesday

Joe, Kenny, and Gimble recorded "Kansas City" and "Prelude to a Kiss" today. Joe is energized when he is playing and recording. He is a professional with Alzheimer's. Joe has never been in a recording studio, but you would never know it.

September 12, 2006—Tuesday

Today was Joe's third recording session, and he played all the great tunes. I love to hear him sing and play. It was just a great night, and I had a front row seat. It was my own private concert with my own faithful Frank Sinatra, only better than Frank.

September 15, 2006—Friday

On the plane to Vegas, Joe kept asking me who invited us to Vegas, what hotel we were staying in, and where we were going to eat. He was very confused. I had a car pick us up at the airport. The driver soon picked up on Joe's condition.

One day I wanted to nap, and Joe was mad. It took me awhile to figure out he wanted me to play all the games with him. He had played poker for over two hours the first day, but then would not play again without me by his side. The last night we were there he went to the room to get our jackets. He was gone for a long time. When he returned to the café, I quizzed him. That was the wrong thing for me to do. Joe said there was construction everywhere. I realized he had turned into the casino instead of the café. He let me have it. He said, "You better not relay any of this to our kids, do you understand?" I felt like I should have answered with a "Yes, Sir."

We saw Don Rickles the next day. On Sunday, Joe had no memory of the show. Then on Monday, he laughed remembering Rickles' jokes.

Oct. 13, 2006—Friday

I had one and a half hours with my Alzheimer's counselor, Howard, and I cried during most of the visit. I told Howard that I was angry with myself for not showing the patience and love Joe deserves. How do I keep a smile on my face when fear is always near?

October 19, 2006

I made myself a schedule for this week. I had many errands, and lots of things I needed to do and things I want to get done. Joe looked at the list and wanted to know what he could do to help. I knew that if

I gave him a job, I would have to walk him through the steps, and I could do it faster on my own. This riled him. Whenever he is irritated with me, he always suggests one of us move out. This gives him the dominant role and puts me on the defense. And it irritates the h— out of me. I have never been the kind of woman who is "quiet and submissive." It's not who I am. Instead, the problem always hangs over us like a mushroom cloud until *I* find a way to dissolve the smoke. From Joe's point of view, I'm the one who always starts the problem. Now with AD, he is not capable of having a conversation or discussion to diffuse the stick of dynamite.

I finally quit trying to dominate the conversation with my point of view. I folded the list of errands, and said nothing more. In a short amount of time, it was forgotten. As I finished each task this week, I had Joe mark off each errand as it was finished. I found this was a way to diffuse the problem. I think he had a feeling of accomplishment.

Oct. 20, 2006

Today, I spent an hour talking to Howard, my Alzheimer's counselor. I think it helped me. I didn't cry as much today. Nothing at home changes from these sessions, but I hear myself go over the problems I am having. By just listening to myself talk aloud, I can usually find a solution to the problems at hand.

Oct. 24, 2006

Today, Dena left three-year-old Drake with us while she went to her hair appointment. Over and over again, Joe asked him his name and age. Drake finally told Joe, "I am *still* Drake and *still* three." I had to laugh. Drake used a tone of voice I try not to use. I felt relieved knowing a three-year-old has a negative reaction after answering the same question over and over. Joe kept asking me whose child Drake was.

October 27, 2006—Friday

I asked Joe if he knew what day it was and if he remembered we are having a party on Saturday to celebrate our fifty-fifth wedding anniversary? He asked if it was someone's birthday. This exchange was played out several times during the day. Surprisingly, he did remember the number of years.

Oct. 28, 2006—Saturday

Joe and I had our fifty-fifth Anniversary party at Casa today. I called off the names of our guests. Joe remembered the names of every spouse. He made a welcome speech, a very good and funny welcoming speech as only Joe can do. He enjoyed the evening—that is, until he got the bill.

Nov. 4, 2006—Saturday

I had only been writing for a short time before Joe began calling me. I didn't use a calm voice when I answered him. I said, "Joe, give me a break. I just came in here to write." He walked to the window opening, and said, "What?" I repeated myself, and he walked away muttering, "Out of sight, out of mind." Then he went outside and began sweeping, showing his disgust.

Nov. 7, 2006—Tuesday

I asked Joe to follow me to the mechanic's to leave my car, but Joe didn't remember where the garage was located. He has no memory of taking our cars to this address. I knew I had to do something to pep him up, so we went to a movie. Joe still enjoys most movies. I hope this doesn't ever change. Going to a movie entertains both of us, and it gets us out of the house.

When I say, "This is no big deal," I realize that it isn't a big deal unless I make it a big deal. And at times, I do make it a big deal if I travel alone without reaching to God for guidance. I know that I must savor every day, and find joy and love upon this journey.

I am responsible for almost everything. Joe still finds pleasure in my cooking, in news on the TV, and in the newspaper he reads over and over during the day. Most of all, he enjoys playing his trumpet. Both my happiness and his happiness rest on my shoulders.

November 5, 2006—Sunday

A lady at church today had on a suit, and I asked her what color it was. Before she could answer, Joe said, "Magenta." I was taken back. I did not know he had ever heard or seen the word *magenta*.

November 20, 2006—Monday

Today, I told Joe that Mindy was driving us to Denton for the North Texas Jazz concert. He was miffed, and responded, emphatically, "I can drive." Then he stared straight at me and, with an edge to his voice, he asked, "What have you told the kids about me? You exaggerate everything. There is nothing wrong with me."

December 14, 2006—Thursday

On the way out of our grandson's choir concert tonight, Ed Burleson asked Joe about the golf game he played today. Joe told Ed he hadn't played golf today. Then when we got home, Joe remembered every hole he had played.

December 16, 2006—Saturday

Joe had a band job this evening at Ridgewood Country Club. I told him the time, that he would eat at the break, and that he was to wear a tuxedo. Sometimes he doesn't absorb this much information. He left murmuring under his breath, "Never will I do this again without getting the information myself." Joe drove to Ridgewood and back home, and remembered where he had parked, I was relieved when I heard the car pull up in the carport, and Joe was hungry when he got home. I made him a sandwich and he had a bowl of ice cream. He didn't remember if he had already eaten.

January 21, 2007—Sunday

Joe was up most of the night with diarrhea. We missed church. He looked over at me before we got out of bed this morning, and said, "When you are with me, I feel better."

His attitude and contentment rest on my meeting each day with a positive attitude. When I ask God to grant me a loving, patient demeanor, I measure up. But if I try to travel the path on my own, I fail.

January 21, 2007—Sunday

If I am quieter than usual, Joe thinks I'm mad and begins his usual dialogue, which is, "I need to get out of here. You are never happy. You're mean. If you don't like it here, then you leave."

My response is always, "Am I not allowed to complain, or to have an opinion?"

He answers, "The way you express yourself is the problem."

If I show any other emotion besides happiness, Joe only knows this way to respond. Discussion for us is useless.

February 3, 20007—Saturday

Jody stopped by for dinner and a visit. He had been to San Marcos to visit Blake and Eric. Dena came over for a visit as well. Joe enjoyed this break in our daily routine. I don't know if our children know how much their visits mean to me. When they visit, it confirms I am not alone on this journey.

February 4, 2007—Sunday

We went to church today. We have missed a lot of Sundays since we got back from Vegas at the end of November.

This week I have had to keep reminding Joe to shower, shave, shampoo, and cut his long fingernails and nose hairs. I have to keep pushing and reminding him. I told him he was not going to walk around looking homeless. I have started laying his clothes out to keep him from wearing the same thing day after day. He loves all this attention. He was the baby of the family, and has been catered to for 78 years. But, of course, he wouldn't agree with that statement.

February 14, 2007—Wednesday

The Burleson's picked us up to go to dinner in West. Ed and Carolyne are so thoughtful to make a point to call, and invite us to dinner often. Joe always enjoys the outings.

Stacy, our granddaughter, dropped by with cookies and candy for us. When she left, Joe called her Roylyn, who is our niece. I don't know where that came from, but it isn't the first time.

February, 17ʼ 2007—Saturday

We met Mindy and the twins for lunch. Joe laughed a lot and made jokes. His humor is priceless. When we got home, he went to the fridge to make a sandwich. He had no memory of our visit with

Mindy and the twins, and had forgotten that he had eaten. He is forgetting more and more that he has eaten.

February 18, 2007—Sunday

Joe didn't know what day it was today. Usually, he writes the date in his checkbook register. Now, before he writes the check, he has already forgotten the date.

We woke up, dressed, and made it to church. Joe visited and talked to lots of folks. He enjoys being with people more than sitting at home with nothing to do.

February 19, 2007—Monday

We are without any schedules, and that is good. It's Presidents' Day, so there's no Rotary. Joe has been zeroed in on Rotary all day. A visit to HEB gave Joe an outing. He was a big help with loading groceries in the car and unloading them at home. His high point for the day was dinner. Sitting down to a meal I prepare always lifts his spirits. It is work for me, and, at times, his glee is irritating. I want to do things for him, but why does it irk me so much? I am tired of taking care of all his needs, especially feeding time—breakfast, lunch, snack time, and dinner. As I read this, I feel I should be ashamed of myself for resenting taking care of the man I love. I ask myself, *WHY?*

March 3, 2007—Saturday

I have said many times that, as wonderful, thoughtful, and good as Joe is, he is somewhat of a prima Donna. Why shouldn't he be? When he was eight or so, Mary Holiday, who had an amateur show every Saturday and a radio show, was impressed with Joe. She would take him to different ladies' clubs for him to sing for them. In Jr. High, his band director was impressed with his musical talent as well. Joe has been in the spotlight from a very young age.

March 5, 2007—Monday

This was a fun and busy day. Joe and I went to church, then Jody and two of our grandsons, Blake and Eric, dropped by for dinner. I made a big bowl of rice, a lot of sautéed chicken, green beans, salad with homemade ranch dressing, rolls, butter, and my famous Johnson tea. For dessert, we had ice cream and the cookies I baked yesterday. Blake and Eric took all that was left back to Dallas plus at least three dozen cookies each. I want to give our grandchildren the same memories our children have—goodies from Gaga's kitchen.

March 6, 2007—Tuesday

Tonight before getting into bed, I put the security alarm on and Joe asked me the code numbers. I said, "I don't remember." A moment later, I finally remembered the right code. He said, "You probably are asking yourself why I want to know the code because I know I'll forget before tomorrow." We had a big laugh.

March 13, 2007—Tuesday

Joe has no idea that today is Barry's birthday. Joe asked me, "Who are the kids and who are their parents?" I hate to come face to face with these kinds of questions, because it makes the reality of this journey real. I know bit by bit, day by day, I am a witness to the disease. Joe still is the same Joe I first met. He loves, is thoughtful, kind, neat, funny, and the epitome of what every wife prays for. But he forgets important dates, forgets any medical problem either of us may have, and just forgets, forgets, forgets. I should always ignore the fact that he forgets, but being human and female, I feel slighted. I know how much he loves me. I know he considers me his best friend. I know I should not feel rejection from him. It is the thief of this disease that robs both of us of these tender years of sharing life together which we have worked long and hard to reach. The sharing of memories or making plans for tomorrow is what I miss the most. If I share a memory with Joe, he forgets it in a short time.

The trick of living with this disease is to accept these facts:

1. Don't expect tomorrow to be better than today.

2. Accept that he will continue to ask the same question over and over.

3. Tomorrow and all days after, he won't remember where to find his glasses, pills, broom, cookies, or the dog food.

4. Just because you set the dog food on the cabinet doesn't mean he'll remember it's for him to feed the dog.

5. If you write a note, he may not remember to check it or even know where the note was placed for him to read.

6. Try your hardest never to say, "I just told you that."

7. Don't expect him to know the way to a familiar location.

8. Don't expect him to remember the names of streets.

9. Anyone with Alzheimer's has very little or no initiative. It is important for you to make plans to keep your loved one stimulated.

10. The burden of being up-beat and happy is on your shoulders. Keeping your tone of voice loving and a smile on your face makes the day brighter.

11. Living in the moment is essential, for the moment is all we may have.

12. These two statements are a must to say aloud each day, "This is no big deal, unless I make it a big deal' and "Joe may have Alzheimer's, but that is not who he is."

April 6, 2007—Friday

We went to the Good Friday church service today. Joe and I discussed his memory problem. "I am glad to be here, and I am not going to worry about it," he told me.

While watching TV, Joe and I admired our Azaleas through the window in full bloom with snowflakes dancing upon the red flowers.

There is not a more loving, attentive man than Joe. He is what every woman prays for, and I am privileged to have him in my life.

April 10, 2007—Tuesday

I am sitting here typing, listening to Joe practice the trumpet. This is a treat. He is playing *It Might As Well Be Spring*. He plays it like no one else, always his own version, simple and jazzy. Who could ask for anything more in life? And so it goes.

April 14, 2007—Saturday

It is cold again today. Texas weather is unpredictable, but never boring until summer.

This morning at breakfast, Joe was reading the paper, and asked, "What did Imus do?" The Imus story has been on the front page in the paper and on all the TV stations most of this week. It isn't that Joe hasn't read about it. He reads the paper from cover to cover from breakfast until bed time. When he asked about Imus this morning, I said in a frustrated voice, "Read the article."

Why do I have this impatient reaction? I find myself, particularly in the morning, building a wall around myself. Why would I want to keep Joe at bay? Why am I cold to his affection in the morning? I have never resisted affection from Joe. I am responsive the rest of the day, but not in the morning. Is this my way of avoiding reality? I have to quiet this urge to push him away. I get irritated when he asks about anything we have just talked about, or that he has read, or something that I know he should know. I don't like myself for having these feelings. I don't want to face the facts. I don't want to see this disease progress. If I don't want to resist his affection, then why do I? His love for me is always prevalent, and he expresses it throughout the day. I never have to wonder if he loves me, because his love for me is obvious. I love him deeply. I love him even with the disease. But I don't love the disease, and I don't love myself when that wall is separating me from him. Why do I act like a spoiled only child? At times, I don't know who I am. I have had to take on more responsibility with appointments, planning outings, keeping up with all the financial decisions, helping Joe look up phone numbers, making out bank deposits, filling out checks, balancing bank statements, while all along trying to include him in all business endeavors. I want to keep him involved and not just put him out to pasture.

April 18, 2007—Wednesday

The more time I spend with him, the better the day is. If I spend much time on the computer, he is lost. I never knew I enjoyed being alone. Now, I see a different me.

April 20, 2007—Friday

I told Joe that I was going to the beauty shop. As I pulled out of the driveway, I asked him if he knew where I was going. He didn't remember. I called home to see if I should bring lunch. His first statement was, "Where are you?" I mentioned lunch, and he said he had already eaten, but couldn't remember eating anything except Fritos. I brought salads home, and he ate most of his.

April 26, 2007—Thursday

Ed, Nick, and Joe played a band job in Temple. I called Luann to tell her that Joe and I were not ignoring them. Joe has repeatedly asked me not to talk about his problem. I didn't want to talk about Joe's memory, even if the rumors are out there. When Joe returned home, I asked him what they had eaten for lunch. He said he didn't eat. I called Carolyne, and she said he had piled up food on his plate, but she didn't know if he had eaten it all.

May 3, 2007—Thursday

Mindy drove us to Dallas to see Dr. Hurd. Joe did seemingly well on some of the questions. His medicine will stay the same. Dr. Hurd asked Joe his opinion about his memory? Joe said he didn't think it was any worse than others his age. Then Dr. Hurd asked me, and I gave a couple examples, "A news article that has been in the paper for weeks is first hand news for Joe each time he reads it. He forgets where his glasses are, but isn't that just a male trait?"

Dr. Hurd laughed, and said, "Maybe."

As Dr. Hurd and I walked down the hallway, I told him that I was upbeat about our visit. He turned to me and said, "You are a strong woman."

I may be strong, but what makes me strong is that I am a woman in love with her man.

May 5, 2007—Saturday

Joe was fixing our coffee this morning, and he asked me again about a news story that has been in the paper for months. I gave some audible negative body language, and Joe immediately began to sing "It Had to Be You." We both cracked up. Words to the song follow:

> *It Had To Be You*
> *It had to be you . . . It had to be you*
> *I wondered around and finally found somebody who*
> *Could make me be true and never be blue.*
> *And make me be glad just to be sad thinking of you.*
> *Some others I've seen, would never be mean,*
> *(began laughing)*
> *Would never be cross or try to be boss,*
> *but they wouldn't do.*
> *For nobody else gave me a thrill*
> *With all your faults I love you still*
> *It had to be you . . . wonderful you*
> *It had to be you*

This is how we meet this disease—with humor and with years of loving each other.

May 12, 2007—Saturday

Joe played for a dance at the Lion's Den. I drove him there, and Ed brought him home. The gig went well. On Sunday, we went to church, which always improves our week.

May 19, 2007—Saturday

I went with Joe to the Shrine dance job. He is at home on the stage more than anywhere else. We had a fun evening.

May 21, 2007—Monday

We stayed home yesterday, because it was raining. Joe doesn't remember it has rained, even though we have been confined to the house for several days.

May 30, 2007—Wednesday

I miss Joe playing golf or having an interest in something. He reads and rereads the paper. I offer to get him a book—something funny—but he is not interested. This devil of a disease destroys any initiative in him. If I make plans or initiate something, he will take part in it. His humor and good nature save us each and every day. Joe never shows any disgust or worries about himself, and that is a daily gift to me.

June 24 2007—Sunday

We are going to a Tea Dance this afternoon. I have told Joe four times today that he knows the honorees who are giving the party. They go to our church and are great dancers, and Joe has complimented them often through the years. But he is completely blank as to who they are, even though he acts like he remembers.

June 29, 2007—Friday

Joe is lazy about shaving. He told me the one thing he misses about working is dressing up. There's not much need to dress up if we stay at home and just piddle in the house and yard.

July 31, 2007—Tuesday

Both Waco families left on vacation today. Joe and I are on our own. I don't see or talk to the girls every day, but knowing they are gone makes me uneasy. I wish the boys spent more time with us. A visit once a month would be nice. I know Joe would enjoy seeing them more often even if he forgets the next day that they were here.

August 11, 2007—Saturday

This is the 37th year for the Band reunion, and it is a sellout once again. Joe greeted the group and remembered most of their names. He played from 7:15p.m. to 11p.m., throwing in a tune or two for me. Despite his disease, he remembers how to play anything and everything—without any sheet music in front of him.

August 17, 2007—Friday

This ol' gal is seventy-seven years old today. My girls gave me a party, and the Waco families were all in attendance. Joe enjoys the family getting together. Nice day.

August 20, 2007—Monday

Joe was lost most of the day. He sat down to his favorite meal, but said he wasn't hungry. He said he felt bad. He usually eats a good dinner even if he isn't hungry. By 8p.m., he was fine and didn't recall that he had felt bad. I couldn't help showing my "Why Do You Do This" side. As hard as I try and pray to always be patient and loving, my unbecoming personality jumps out. It is so hard to accept this disease. I am trying to keep calm, with a loving persona, but at times the love and calm escape me. It is hard for me to comprehend that Joe truly cannot remember things. He doesn't even remember that he forgets! Some of the time I forget that he doesn't remember that he forgets. Try to figure that one out. I will manage to walk in love and to appreciate and celebrate each day. It is so easy to love this guy. It is my shortcomings that get in the way.

August 31, 2007—Friday

I think I have everything ready for our trip to Europe. I even have my Swiss Francs and Euros in a zippered case, and I have money designated for the bus driver and tour director. I am ready. Four more days, and we are off.

September 5, 2007—Wednesday

Hold onto your seat. This next week reads like a disaster novel. On this trip I was exposed to the Sun Downing of Alzheimer's. Sun downing can be either hallucination or delusional conduct. I call it the "Al zone." It can last an hour or several hours.

We were late leaving Waco because of a bad thunderstorm. Joe wanted to get off the plane. I kept thinking that things would improve when we arrived in Dallas. Joe finally calmed down, and we boarded our plane at DFW and were on our way to JFK in New York. When we arrived at JFK airport to make our connection, I had ordered assistance to take us to our gate. I sat down in the wheelchair, and our gate was directly across from where we exited the plane. I felt pretty silly being pushed across the hallway.

We had great seats on the next plane, and were off to Zurich. At this time, Joe was fine. He had a couple of beers, and after a while we ordered dinner. Joe suddenly thought we were on a bus, and he was worried that the rain would cave in the ceiling of the bus. I explained to him many times that we were on a plane going to Switzerland, but nothing I said penetrated his thoughts. He was certain we were on a bus with rain beating on the ceiling, and he would ask over and over, "Who are all these people, and where did you meet them?" He thought they were politicians and that I knew who they were.

On one of many trips to the potty, Joe left his passport in the bathroom. A hostess kindly returned it. Joe would not take a nap, and he loudly kept saying sexual things and asking too many questions. This went on for the entire eight-hour trip.

September 6, 2007—Thursday

We arrived in Zurich, Switzerland at 7 a.m. Joe began looking for a bathroom. I saw a nearby sign directing us to toilets for *Men, Women* and *Handicapped.* Joe headed toward one of the three doors, and entered the women's door. I waited and waited, and he finally came out without his passport around his neck. I looked in the bathroom, and he had dropped it in the potty.

Joe was very confused about the airport setting. We finally found the luggage rack, and it was empty. Our luggage had been lost. Joe was certain our luggage was still on the plane. "We don't know where the plane is," I told him. When I sat down to make a claim on our luggage, Joe would not cooperate. He said, "That boy has our luggage stashed in the back room." I tried to calm Joe down. The young man on the computer located one piece of luggage still at JFK, and said the other may be in Germany. All the while, Joe kept telling me that this guy knew where our luggage was. I kept trying to talk to the agent while assuring Joe that everything was fine. Finally, the agent said our luggage would be delivered to the hotel.

When we finally arrived to our hotel room about 8 a.m., I was ready for a nap, but Joe wasn't tired. He wanted to go back to the Air Terminal and look for our luggage. I begged him to get in bed and rest, but he said he was going to get in the car and drive home. I said, "Joe, we don't have a car, and 'Home' is on the other side of the

Atlantic. We're in Zurich, Switzerland right now." The phrase "Zurich, Switzerland" never registered in his mind, and he informed me in his judicial voice that he had driven to Waco from Houston many times.

Our luggage arrived at the hotel that afternoon. I figured Joe sun downed all the way from Dallas to Zurich, and was still sun downing several hours after we checked in to the hotel.

September 8, 2007—Saturday

At breakfast, there was a group of twelve guys eating near us. As it turned out, they were musicians from England, and they were there to perform a concert. I introduced Joe to them, including a litany of Joe's achievements. After Joe stopped being embarrassed, he visited with the group. Joe is much shyer than I have ever been.

At dinner, we joined our tour and went downtown for a tour of the city and dinner. Before leaving the hotel, we met a gentleman named Howard. He was very nice, but talked a lot. At the restaurant, Joe had to go to the men's room, and I asked Howard to assist him to make sure he found his way back to the group. Howard picked up on Joe's condition, and that gave me comfort.

Tomorrow we begin our bus tour of Switzerland. After that, our next stop will be the south of France, ten days in Paris, and a return trip to La Rochelle and Fouras, France where we lived in 1952. Waco will be the last leg of our final trip to Europe.

September 9, 2007—Sunday

We boarded the bus for our first day in Switzerland. The scenery from the bus was amazing. Everywhere we looked was like a picture from a book. Beauty surrounded us. We reached the uppermost destinations in the Alps and had a few minutes off the bus to feel and smell the air. The temperature was about 31 degrees, and mounds of snow were everywhere. Joe enjoyed the mountains.

Today's trip was everything I've always imagined Switzerland to be.

When we arrived back to our room, Joe was restless. He wanted to know what we were going to do the next day. I told him, and he was worried that I was sneaking away to ski with some of the men on our tour. I tried telling him no one was going skiing, but he didn't buy it. He kept saying, "Why are you going skiing? You don't know how, and you might get hurt."

We had dinner just the two of us. We went back to the room, and Joe again started questioning why I wanted to go skiing. He said he was going to drive home. I was so stressed, because I had eaten very little and had slept with only one eye open since leaving Waco four days before.

I knew I should listen to my body and not worry about finishing the trip. I went to the lobby, and had the desk clerk pull up American Airlines on their computer to see if we could get a return ticket to DFW on September 14th. They had two Business class nonstop tickets to DFW on the 14th. We would have to go back to Zurich to catch the plane home. Here we were in the Swiss mountains changing hotels every night, and I was clueless as to how to get confirmation on a return ticket on the 14th before canceling our return ticket on the 23rd from Paris. I decided to call our travel agent in Waco to make the change for us. We went to bed, and I planned on getting up at 3a.m., thinking that the travel agent would be in the office back in America at that time. I called several times, and finally realized that it was 8p.m. Sunday night in Waco and not 10a.m. Monday morning. With that realization, I could sleep a few hours.

At breakfast, I told Joe I was going to go talk with Leslie, our tour director. There was this lady from upstate NY who had joined us for breakfast and as I began to get up she said to me in her NY accent, "Sit down, and let Leslie have breakfast in peace." I shot her a look, went to Leslie's table, and asked for help exchanging our tickets. I filled Leslie in on our previous few days, and she said, "Don't worry. I'll take care of it."

We boarded the bus and had another gorgeous scenic trip through the mountains and gorges. The scenery is something I can't describe. We stopped for lunch at a quaint restaurant gift shop. At this stop, Leslie informed me that she had talked to the London office and as soon as we arrived in Lugano, Italy she would take us to see a doctor for evaluation. The doctor needed to observe how disoriented Joe was, and also my stress level, in order to insure us getting a partial refund on our Switzerland tour.

Leslie told the doctor I was having heart palpitations, which wasn't true at all. The nurse took my blood pressure (120/70), and my pulse (60). The doctor said, "Very good." My stress was showing through my tremor, and I was shaking badly. The doctor asked Joe where he was, and Joe replied, "Georgetown, Texas, of course." Leslie and the doctor went in his office and had a conference with London. Leslie was working on getting us tickets back to the States on September 11th. That was music to my ears.

Sure, I wanted to finish this last trip to Europe, but my intuition was telling me to get back to Texas. Was it my intuition or was this a message from God? Looking back, I had been up for days, never letting Joe leave my side. I wasn't in any mental condition to make a decision. I know it was God. Leslie came to our room before dinner, and told us she had made arrangements for our departure the next day from Lugano, Switzerland at 6:30a.m. to Zurich on September 11th.

I called Mindy to have one of them pick us up at DFW and call our travel agent. Mindy asked if I knew what Tuesday was. I said, "Yes, it's the anniversary of the 9/11 attacks. Don't worry about it. We're coming home, and we'll get there safely." The travel time was estimated at thirteen hours from Lugano to Zurich, and on to Dallas. I found a jazz guitarist on the head set for Joe to listen to on the plane, and he was content for all thirteen hours.

September 12, 2007—Wednesday

After we made it through customs back in Texas, Jody was waiting for us. We climbed in his car, and were in Waco by 6p.m. Sunny, our house sitter, had meat loaf, mashed potatoes, broccoli, and chicken salad made for us. Joe was so happy to be home. Jody stayed for a while and left for Dallas about 8p.m.

After playing with Holly, watching TV, and walking around outside, Joe and I went to bed about 10:30p.m. I was so happy to get off the roller-coaster ride I had been on for a full week. I decided there would be no more plane trips for Joe and I unless two of our children were traveling with us. That was more stress than one person should go through alone.

September 20, 2007—Thursday

Joe was diagnosed with Alzheimer's four years ago in November. This morning was the first time Joe has called me Iva. He thought I was his sister, Iva Belle. He asked me if I had seen any of my old friends from Kansas where Iva and Lyle lived. I kept telling him I was his wife, Deane, but he still thought I was Iva. This went on for an hour or more. I was hurt, frightened, and felt like I had hit a brick wall. I made a decision to go talk with our minister, Jimmie Johnson, with my Alzheimer's counselor, Howard, and also to make an appointment with a psychiatrist. I needed all three.

September 23, 2007—Sunday

Today was the day we were supposed to return from Europe. I am fine having missed the rest of Switzerland, the South of France, Nice, and Paris, jazz clubs, upscale dinners, and our last visit to Fouras, France. I am sure there will come a time when I am sorry we had to cut the trip to six days, but under the circumstances, that was the only option. Even today, I would not plan another trip anywhere with Joe in his condition.

We went to church this morning, then celebrated Mindy's 50th birthday party at the Elite. The whole family was there. It was very festive and enjoyable. Our daughter Mindy is a beautiful fifty.

September 24, 2007—Monday

Thoughts from me to Mindy:

Time doesn't stand still, memories expand, love grows, and families move on. Grandchildren warm our hearts and give us a glimpse into the future, our mates grow dearer, and we lean on our adult children more, knowing that we can.

Life is truly a journey. At these Crossroads, I am content. I count my blessings knowing that things could be more stressful and may be on down the road. I am learning to live in the moment. I am blessed to be the wife of your dad. I don't just love him. I am in love with him and have been since that remarkable night and our first kiss on December 31, 1950. There is a difference between loving someone and being in love with them.

I am the mother of two handsome and thoughtful sons, and two beautiful, caring daughters.

I have it all. May you find this love and joy I enjoy every day!

Love,
Mother

September 26, 2007—Wednesday

Dena brought Colby and Drake over to stay with Joe and me. Joe played outside with them for a short period. He has been more content ever since we returned home from Europe.

September 28, 2007—Friday

I met with Howard, and told him about the stress of our trip, how confused Joe was, and that I had hit a brick wall.

October 4, 2007—Thursday

We had our yearly checkup with Dr. Browder. Joe and I both got an A+ rating even with my sick stiff legs, bad knees, tremor, and Joe with his memory loss. Joe is healthy in every way except for those damn "tangles" clogging up the blood vessels in his brain. We all must play with the cards dealt to us. Joe doesn't remember my tremor or stiff legs from one day to the next. It isn't intentional, or that he doesn't care. It is what it is.

October 5, 2007—Friday

I waited until Joe closed the gates before I left to go get my hair fixed. As he was closing the last gate, a shrub caught Joe's eye. Once I was out of sight, Joe got his trimmers, and the Abellia was no longer safe. When I came home, Joe was hurriedly filling a garbage can with debris, but on a second look Joe had whittled down a shoulder high pink blooming Abellia to about 2 feet. I was upset, to say the least. I don't know what makes him cut bushes even when the bush is in full bloom. I have had to nag in order to keep him from trimming the crepe Myrtles which are in full bloom. I need to remember that he doesn't remember.

October 6, 2007—Saturday

Joe is playing in a band with his friend, Aubrey, tonight at the Lion's Den. I took him there, and Aubrey brought him home. Joe was upbeat when he got home. Music is Joe. Joe is music.

October 18, 2007—Thursday

We were in bed tonight, and Joe said he could not place me in his mind. He could see Nick and Ed, but not me. I turned on the light so he could see me, but for some reason he couldn't get a picture of me in his mind. After a while, he said he could picture me in his head.

Excerpt from the book "*36-Hour Day*":

People with dementing illnesses may lose their ability to recognize things or people, not because they have forgotten them or because their eyes are not working but because the brain is not able to put together information properly. This is called agnosia from Latin meaning "to not know." It can be a baffling symptom.

October 26, 2007—Friday

I saw Dr. Grayson today, and he thought he was telling me things about Alzheimer's that I didn't know. His dad had AD. I know he wants to help, but that is impossible. Joe has Alzheimer's, and it is something we must learn to live with.

October 28, 2007—Sunday

Jimmie Johnson called Joe several weeks ago to play and sing at our church for an interdenominational celebration for families of Alzheimer's. The girls came, and for two hours we all listened to family members of Alzheimer's patients relate only doom and gloom while talking about their loved ones. The girls kept asking me why I let Joe attend the "Celebration of Life" service. I told them not to worry, because Joe would not remember all the doom and gloom testimonials.

Joe on the trumpet and Kenny on guitar were last on the program, and it was a long program. Joe was supposed to play and sing 'Skylark' and 'Stardust.' But as they were going up the steps, Joe said, "Kenny, let's play 'Back Home Again in Indiana,' and then get the hell out of here." This is a favorite of jazz players.

I learned something important that day. I learned to bury the negatives of this journey and glorify the positives. Not one speaker spoke about accomplishments and dreams of their loved one. In the two hours of the program, not one relative of the Alzheimer's person spoke of anything except the last days of their life and how hurt they were when the relative didn't remember them. If I ever find myself speaking about Joe and this journey we are on, I will shout from the rooftops that this man's personality, his love of family, his talents, and accomplishments, all outweigh Alzheimer's. I'll leave out the sadness, because his life involves more love, talents, and friendships than it does sad stories.

P.S. Today is our 56th wedding Anniversary. We went to Casa to celebrate.

October 31, 2007—Wednesday

Joe always enjoys handing out candy on Halloween night. Dena and her brood came by to trick or treat, and it was a joy for both Joe and I.

November 2, 2007—Friday

Before I left the house today, I put a note on Joe's wrist so he would know where I was. When I finished my errands, I came by the house to pick up Joe to go to Burger King. On the way to lunch, he said, "I didn't know where you went." Joe spent the day sweeping again.

November 3, 2007—Saturday

I was watching a show in bed, and Joe didn't like the TV being on. When I questioned him, he became angry and said, "This is my house, and I make the rules." This conversation went on for a while, and then he asked, "Where is my wife?" At that moment, I realized he thought he was in bed with someone else. I turned on the lights, and after about twenty minutes he was fine. Another learning experience—don't be defensive until I know what he is thinking or imagining.

November 5, 2007—Monday

I cooked dinner tonight, and Joe said I was not doing my part around the house. I defended myself, but that does not solve anything for Joe. It doesn't matter that I made breakfast, went to the grocery store, lifted weights, and heated up the roast with salad and rolls for dinner. Shortly after, he had forgotten he was mad at me, and we were back to normal—whatever that is.

November 6, 2007—Tuesday

Today, I had my first appointment with Dr. Sawyer (psychiatrist). I told him about our trip to Switzerland, and Joe's sun downing. The doctor prescribed 5 mg. of Lexapro daily. I hope it will stop my flow of tears.

November 9, 2007 Friday

Joe was reading about an Air show out of town. I am not a fan of air shows, but I will go with him tomorrow if he even remembers it. Joe swept leaves most of the day. He played a dance job this evening. He looks forward to all his band jobs. When he plays his trumpet, he is Joe the music man.

November 10, 2007 Saturday

First thing Joe said before he got up was, "I don't care that much about the Air Show." I was boggled that he remembered about the Air Show, and yet he can't remember the names of his grandkids or even where he keeps his underwear.

November 11, 2007 Sunday

Today was a normal Sunday. We went to church, I cooked a roast, and Joe put out the trash. With Joe sweeping every day, we have lots of trash.

November 19, 2007 Monday

Joe kept asking me if he had been paid for the band job Friday night, so I called Ed who said that they had been paid. I checked Joe's tux, and the money was in his pocket. We went to the bank to cash his check.

I need to buy a new door knob for the back door, because Joe keeps locking himself out. I have to figure something out so that he can't lock himself out during the day.

Tommy Letbetter, Joe's cousin, called, and I told him about Joe. It upset Tommy. He is coming for a visit in January.

November 22, 2007—Thursday

Today is Thanksgiving. Mindy had dinner for all of us. Joe was sitting next to Barry watching TV, and Joe didn't know whose house he was in.

November 27, 2007—Tuesday

Today is Joe's 79th Birthday. I told Dr. Sawyer I did not take his last prescription. I don't need it. I have my confidence back, though tears surfaced when I mentioned my mother's name.

November 30, 2007—Friday

I put a note on Joe's wrist with a rubber band before I left for the beauty shop, but he forgot it was on his wrist. I have left notes on the bulletin board, on the bar, taped to the back door, and on his wrist, but. . . "out of sight—out of mind."

December 3, 2007—Monday

Today, Joe said, "I can't do anything anymore." I understand his frustration. He doesn't see what needs to be done, forgets where things are, and has trouble keeping up with the time and days of the week.

December 4, 2007—Tuesday

The twins put our Christmas tree up, and put everything back up. After they finished the tree, the boys decorated the outside. Our grandsons are thoughtful and loving boys. It is a treat to have grandchildren old enough and with the desire to help Joe and me.

December 13, 2007—Thursday

Often times, I want my own space where I don't have to talk to Joe, but that is not the way you treat anyone, especially the person you love who is having memory problems. Joe needs love and interaction to feel secure and safe.   Joe swept leaves most of the day.

December 15, 2007—Saturday

I have a hard time getting Joe to shower and shave. Tonight he told me emphatically that he would decide when to bathe.

Joe has a different look in his eyes some days—like he is pissed, lost, and unsure of himself. I said, "Joe quit wandering through the house." He replied, coldly, "Like a mental patient?"

Later, I was talking to one of our kids on the phone, and Joe asked me, "How much money does it cost for you to call the kids?" If this is a new stage where he is going to continually bug me about talking on the phone, it is going to be a trying time.

P.S. Joe was restless, walking and pacing most of the night.

December 31, 2007—Monday

Fifty-seven years ago tonight, Joe asked if he could kiss me Happy New Year, and you know the rest of the story. Tonight we stayed awake, waiting for our New Year's kiss.

January 6, 2008—Sunday

Joe said he was going to get a burger, and he didn't need for me to go with him. I told him I would ride without giving him directions, but he still didn't know where to go. I asked him what he was going to order, and he said a burger. I then said something that made him mad, and he told me to get out of the car. I stayed put and stayed quiet. By the time we returned home, he had forgotten about the verbal exchange.

January 7, 2008—Monday

Joe needs a lot of attention. He would say that statement is false, but I can tell he is upbeat when he gets a lot of attention. Because he was the youngest in his family growing up, he has had a lot of attention since birth.

P.S. All the different effects that Alzheimer's may have on Joe will never mask the man Joe is.

January 14, 2008—Monday

AD victims have no incentive. If an idea pops into their head, it is forgotten in minutes. I need to remember this truth, and not criticize Joe. I just don't understand how one minute a person can hear something, and in the bat of an eye the thought is vanished from their memory.

I must start saying the Serenity prayer every night and throughout the day.

God, give me the serenity to accept the things I can't change,
The courage to change the things I can,
And the wisdom to know the difference.

January 19, 2008—Saturday

Joe played a band job tonight. I think it is good for him to get out without me and do something with the guys. He has been looking forward to the job. When Evan called out "I Thought about You," the guys didn't know if Joe could remember the tune without a fake book, but he played the hell out of the song—bridge and all. My Joe does not need a fake book ever. Joe and I need a cure for Alzheimer's.

January 22, 2008—Tuesday

For dinner, I reheated the rice, filets, and cornbread. Joe sat at the bar for a while, and when he joined me he asked me where Jody and Barry went. I told him that no one had been here but us. He said, "Isn't this what happens before the end?"

February 15, 2008—Friday

Today, I told Dr. Moreledge I wanted to have the Deep Brain Stimulation surgery (DBS) to control my tremor. I will have my head shaved, the Surgeon will drill two holes in my head—one for the left hand and one for the right hand. I will be awake the entire time. One week later, an instrument will be inserted right below my collar bone, the wires under my scalp will be connected to the instrument and I will be able to turn the battery powered instrument off or on which will control my tremor.

February 19, 2008—Tuesday

Joe got up early and asked, "Who is dead?" We had soup for lunch, and then picked up acorns in the yard. Joe took Holly for a walk, and we had barbecue chicken for dinner. I am keeping my fingers crossed that this new Exelon patch Dr. Moreledge gave us will stall Joe's Alzheimer's in its tracts.

March 8, 2008—Saturday

Barry came by for a visit, but Joe didn't talk much. I think when there is a lot of talk he has a hard time following the conversation. Joe loved seeing Barry.

March 10, 2008—Monday

I think the Exelon patches may work. Nick is having surgery tomorrow, and I suggested that Joe call and wish him luck. He said he would call later. About an hour later, Joe asked what their phone number was. He not only remembered to call, but he also remembered why he was calling.

March 11, 2008—Tuesday

Mindy took me to Austin to see Dr. Patel, who will perform my Deep Brain Stimulation surgery, and yes, it scares me.

March 13, 2008—Thursday

Today is Barry's fifty-second Birthday. I miss being with our kids on their special day.

Every day when Joe fixes my coffee, he asks the same question, "How much sugar?" I answer, "I don't use sugar." This conversation takes place daily.

March 24, 2008—Monday

Joe asked again about his mom, wanting to know if she had a will or any money. I explained it again. He told me that he felt sorry for me fooling with an old forgetful man, and he wouldn't blame me if I left him. Dealing with Joe is a lot like dealing with an oversized two-year-old. He can't help that he forgets, and I must remember this at all times. Joe is still the same person with good manners, a loving disposition, talents, and morals. Only, now he has a memory problem.

March 29, 2008—Saturday

Joe has no memory of seeing the Four Freshman last night in Fort Worth. This is hard for me to believe. Joe and I first heard the Four Freshmen with Stan Kenton in May 1953 in New York at Bird Land. This group has been his favorite for years, and now he has forgotten overnight that he saw them in concert less than 24 hours ago. I must learn to be satisfied in the moment.

April 8, 2008—Tuesday

I had my left cataract removed. This surgery seemed longer than the last one. Joe was not happy that he stayed at home when I had my first cataract surgery, so this time he went with us. When I asked him if he wanted to come, he said, "I am your husband." He realizes that he was the one to lead in the past, and he still wants to do it. I wish it was that easy.

This week has been a roller coaster ride. Joe has called me Iva three nights this week. When it happened the second night, I had a mild melt down. I cried and finally got him to understand how it made me feel. He said he would feel the same way. I told him it was crazy for me to be jealous of a dead woman. These spells of sun downing last from fifteen minutes to hours. I am left with a sadness I must overcome. When Joe sun downs, he is not himself.

April 14, 2008—Monday

When getting on the elevator today, a gentleman stepped out, and Joe called him by name—Otho Neeley. I was shocked Joe remembered his name. I bet Joe didn't see Otho twice a year when Joe was working at the Court House, and yet Joe knew his name immediately.

P.S. Last Thursday, before we went to bed, I could sense that Joe did not know who I was. As we were making the bed, Mindy called and Joe told her that he and his sister were making the bed. This really gets to me.

He showered, and when he got in bed, I was Iva again to him. I was not kind about it, and when I asked him how he would react if it was me calling him another man's name, he said it would bother him. In about thirty minutes, I was Deane to him again.

April 23—Wednesday

We attended the bank cookout today, and Joe stayed very close to me. Our friend, Bill Beazely, came over to talk with us. I knew he wanted to ask how Joe was doing but felt uncomfortable. His wife died with AD. He encouraged me to take care of myself and to get lots of help.

April 27, 2008—Sunday

Joe thought I was Iva again today while we were driving around town. About 45 minutes later, he knew who I was and said he could understand my reaction. He said he didn't know how or why his mind did that.

April 29, 2008—Tuesday

The following is a letter I wrote to Dr. Morledge:

Dear Dr. Morledge,
I don't feel right discussing Joe's digression in front of him. I try to encourage Joe and to be caring, but I'm not always thoughtful.
Here are the perks Joe has shown while wearing the patch:

1. *If the dog bowls are empty, he fills them.*
2. *One day, I gave him instructions to do more than one thing. I thought to myself, "More than one thing is too much." But Joe completed all three tasks.*
3. *I suggested Joe call a friend about his surgery. Thirty minutes passed, and Joe asked for the phone number and remembered why he was calling.*
4. *He is neat, and likes to match his socks with his shirt.*
5. *When he hears me rattling dishes because of my tremor, he comes in the kitchen to help.*
6. *He makes up the bed most mornings and always wipes out the sink after he shaves.*
7. *He unloads the dishwasher, and knows where most of the dishes belong.*
8. *After our meals, he wipes the table.*
9. *He has played three band jobs in the past six weeks, and remembers all the songs by ear.*
10. *He is always thoughtful, appreciative of all I do, and his sense of humor is always present.*

The Alzheimer's is prevalent daily, and he still asks the same question multiple times. At times I think I have a 79-year old that is no more than two. He has called me his sister's name a lot lately. He looks right at me but cannot see me, because, in his brain, I am Iva. I know it is foolish to be jealous of a dead woman, but at times that jealousy-demon emerges. When he calls me Iva, I tell him, "I am not Iva, I am your lover." That usually does the trick.

He can't recall the names of his grandchildren, but remembers the names of his close friends. This is a challenge.

I am traveling a path with bumps of anxiety, fear, and the unknown. But the journey is littered with lots of love and hope. The two sentences I repeat daily are: 1. Joe has Alzheimer's disease, but that is not who he is. 2. It is no big deal unless I make it a big deal.

We will see you on Wednesday May 7ʰ.

Sincerely,
Deane Johnson

May 4, 2008—Sunday

Joe drove home from church, and hit the rear view mirror coming in the gate. He heard it, but by the time he got out of the car, he had forgotten he hit it. We talked about it, and I told him he should let me drive. His answer was, "I am not ready to give up that part of my life." I told him I had to give up acrobatics. He didn't think that was funny.

May 7, 2008—Wednesday

Mindy picked Joe and me up at 8:15a.m. to go to Austin. Dr. Morledge took him off the patch and prescribed Exelon 3mg pills twice a day. Joe was allergic to the patch.

May 9, 2008—Friday

I made a run to the grocery store this afternoon. Joe unloaded the groceries to bring into the house. While the car door was open, our dog Holly jumped into the car. Joe didn't see her do it. After putting up the groceries and getting ready to eat, we began to wonder where Holly was. We looked everywhere. I thought maybe we had closed her up in the store room. I went out to check, and there she was in the back seat of the car, hot as a firecracker. I don't think Joe ever understood the danger Holly was in. A lesson I learned: always check the car after Joe unloads the groceries.

May 19, 2008—Monday

This morning when Joe was measuring my coffee, he asked if I wanted sugar in mine. "No," I answered, as I do every day. He quickly retorted with, "Get your ass up, and fix it yourself." He doesn't remember I have a tremor, and when your husband of fifty-six years remembers nothing about you, it hurts. He turned to walk away, and I screamed at him, "Don't you care enough about me to remember I have a tremor?" At that, he turned with fist clinched. I told him if he ever hit me, I would throw him out of the house. Thirty minutes later, he didn't remember what had happened.

May 21, 2008—Wednesday

I just found out that Leland, a longtime friend, has died. We were neighbors for twelve years,

May 22, 2008—Thursday

Mindy and I took dinner to the Colliers. Joe went with us, and we visited for about an hour. Joe had forgotten that it was Leland who had died. He quickly made a joke to cover up his memory loss.

May 24, 2008—Saturday

Joe played a job at the Karem Temple tonight. When he stood up to sing, play his trumpet, and talk to the audience, he came to life. Joe's home is not here or at the Court House, but on the stage, playing and singing.

May 28, 2008—Wednesday

Joe accused me of going behind his back to hire the painters. He forgot he had made the deal with them. I get so flustered trying to defend myself without being harsh. Joe is not happy this week.

May 30, 2008—Friday

Linda, my hair dresser, always asks how things are going at home. Today, I told her I had to learn how to accept the stage Joe is in at the present, because it could be worse this time next year. I explained that I would miss out on today if I whined about the circumstances. What was Joe like a year ago? I don't think he is that much more forgetful than he was last year.

June 13, 2008—Friday

Joe cried this morning. He dreamed his mother had died. He wanted to know about the arrangements. I assured him that when she died, he had made the arrangements and attended her funeral. Joe was relieved knowing he did this for his mother.

June 15, 2008—Sunday

Today, Joe asked me if any of his family members are still living.

June 17, 2008—Tuesday

I finally got Joe to shower today. Last night he told me he had showered, but I knew he hadn't. He thought he had pulled one on me, but I had washed all the white clothes, and Joe had no shorts in the empty hamper. He didn't take his pills last night either. I have to stay on top of him to make sure he takes his pills, showers, and shaves.

June 20, 2008—Friday

I was working on my journal on the computer today, and Joe thought I was talking to someone. He wanted to see what I was doing. I have never been in a chat room, and I didn't even know Joe knew what it was.

P.S. Joe hid his wallet again last night, and I found it under some clothes and boxes in the bedside table this afternoon. Life isn't monotonous.

June 21, 2008—Saturday

Today began in harmony and satisfaction. Joe and I were at home until I took him to the Clifton House to play a band job. He was upbeat and looking forward to the night. I had an uneventful but calm evening until I received a call from Carolyne that Joe was mad and would not ride home with Ed or Kenny. Joe was upset because the host wanted the band to repeat the Cotton Eyed Joe again and again. Everyone was dancing and rowdy. Joe was sitting on the front row floor level and was afraid that someone might fall on him and make him hurt his lips. He has always been protective of his lips, because his lips are his livelihood while playing a trumpet. Joe was more than ready to pack up the horn and quit.

When he returned home, he felt badly about saying mean things to Ed. I think Joe had a good reason to get up from his chair, but not to say hurtful words to a good friend. Later, Ed dropped by to bring Joe his mouth piece case, and Joe apologized to Ed.

June 22, 2008—Sunday

We missed church again. We were tired and stressed from last night's fiasco. Joe never mentioned the incident that transpired last night. He has no memory of the job or of what happened between him and Ed.

June 28, 2008—Saturday

At dinner, Joe asked where the kids went that were playing in the back yard. He said that he waved at them. He keeps thinking someone is here besides us. The sun downing lasted less than an hour.

July 1, 2008—Tuesday

Joe tells me every night that I belong just to him. But tonight, Joe told me I belonged to the whole world. He is a loving husband. He compliments me daily, and tells me often that I make good decisions. I hope I always make the best decisions for the two of us, which would be to keep Joe by my side till death do us part.

July 2, 2008—Wednesday

Our grandsons, Jackson and Eric, were fertilizing my flower bed, and Joe didn't realize they were our grandsons. Joe thought I had hired strangers to do major work, and that I had not consulted him before hiring them. Finally he came back to the present.

July 7, 2010—Monday

Joe went with Mindy and I to the beauty shop to get my buzz cut for my Deep Brain Surgery. I dreaded getting my head shaved, but I look better than I expected.

Jody is staying here with Joe until we return from Austin. Joe is not happy that Jody will be staying with him, but there is no way I could leave Joe alone.

Dena and Mindy picked me up at 5p.m. to go to Austin. We ate at the Cheese Cake Factory. On the way to the hotel we saw a double rainbow, and our room number was 316. A double rainbow is good luck, and John 3:16 is a Bible verse we all know. These were omens.

July 8, 2008—Tuesday

I checked into the hospital at 6a.m. today in order to prepare for my Deep Brain Stimulation surgery tomorrow. Dr. Patel came into my room at noon. A nurse had shaved my head, but Dr. Patel shaved it closer. I then realized that the time had come for him to put five screws in my head. The doctor cut my scalp, scraped a little on my skull and then he brought out the screws and drill. It was a battery-powered drill. The screws needed to be tweaked, so they got a small sterilized screw driver after they had used the drill. Mindy and Dena got cornered in the room and watched it from the beginning until the end. My head was wrapped in gauze to help cushion the screws so I might sleep tonight. Dr. Patel asked me if I wanted something for pain, and I said I was fine. Both girls chimed in and said, yes, give her something for pain. We were back in the hotel by 3p.m. I did have a difficult time finding a comfortable way to sleep on a pillow.

July 9, 2008—Tuesday

This is the big day. I have been going over this operation in my mind for two months. When I was rolled to the OR, I began to cry. I wasn't crying because of fear, I was crying because Joe wasn't with me. He has been with me every time I have gone to the hospital for the past fifty-six years. Mindy and Dena were by my side though, which was a comfort, but I was missing the only person in my life who had provided me with security and the comfort that I needed. This is one aspect of Alzheimer's that is particularly hard on me. A wife needs her husband, and a husband needs his wife in trying times. It was a lonely ride to the OR.

July 10, 2008—Wednesday

I was released from ICU late this afternoon. I talked to Joe. His voice was music to my ears and better than any pain pill. Joe had called Jody "Tommy" all week. Tommy is Joe's cousin and Joe's only living relative. Joe told me they had eaten out every meal and that Tommy (Jody) was spending a lot of money. Joe and I talked for some time on the phone. He told me how much he missed me and that he had worried about me. Joe didn't miss me any more than I missed him.

July 11, 2008—Friday

The girls and I got back to Waco around 3p.m. Joe was glad to see me, and he had no idea how glad I was to see him. Jody said Joe remembered that I was coming home today, and that Joe got up and showered and shaved without any prodding. Jody also said Joe was mad most of the week, saying he didn't understand why I had been at the mall so long. Jody said he repeatedly told Joe where I was and that they marked the days off the calendar until it was the day I was to come home.

July 14, 2008—Monday

Mindy and I went back to Austin for my final surgery. Dena stayed with Joe.

Mindy and I had dinner at I-Hop. While we were eating, I noticed a big burly guy with dark, penetrating eyes looking at me. He walked over to our table, and he told Mindy and I that he felt a strong spirit coming from our table. He told us he had been in Iraq, that he was adopted, and that he takes care of his parents. He praised Mindy for her kindness, saying "Family is everything." We shook his hand, he bid us farewell, and was gone as quickly as he appeared. Was he an Angel? I think he was. We checked into room 316 again for the night.

July 15, 2008—Tuesday

The surgery went well today. I was late getting out of the hospital, which put us late getting back to Waco. Mindy spent the night again.

I went to bed early. Joe and Mindy stayed up to watch TV. I heard Mindy explaining to Joe that she was Mindy, his daughter. The sound of Mindy's voice startled me. I know how frightening it is when Joe doesn't recognize you, so I got up and went into the TV room. I told Joe over and over that Mindy was our daughter. He said again and again, "This can't be right."

Mindy explained that she felt like Joe was coming on to her. This was her father, and he didn't know it. Joe went into a rant about how we love different people in different ways such as mother-daughter, husband-wife, and friend–friend. Mindy called Jim, her husband, to come over. Joe could sense that something was wrong, but he didn't know what the problem was. Joe looked at Jim and said, "If I did something wrong, I'm sorry." Joe didn't know what was going on with Mindy crying, and Jim coming over at 11p.m. Mindy was upset, Joe was upset, and I was confused and upset but I had to comfort both my daughter and my husband.

We all went to bed in separate bedrooms. Joe wanted me by his side in our bed. Mindy was in the other bedroom crying. I spent the next couple of hours going from one room to the other feeling a need to comfort my daughter who had just experienced her father not knowing who she was while making a pass at her, and Joe needed me to comfort him because he was so confused about what happened. He didn't know why Jim was here, why Mindy was crying, and why I was jumping from one room to the other. I wished I could have been in two places at the same time. Both Joe and Mindy needed me.

Joe, an overly protective father and husband, outstanding citizen, retired Judge, who is well known, loved and admired, is the Joe we all know. Alas, Joe-with-Alzheimer's was present tonight.

July 17, 2008—Thursday

Mindy stayed at her home last night. It is going to take some time for her to move past this trauma. Joe has no memory of last night. He would be horrified if he remembered. Damn this disease.

July 25, 2008—Friday

Mindy drove Joe and I to Austin to have Dr. Morledge program my battery implant. Because of my surgery and this new battery, I don't have a tremor in either hand. Tonight, we met Mindy's family at I-Hop, and I was the center of attention. I ate with a fork, I put on lipstick, I could write, and I didn't need a straw to drink my water. My life has improved 100%, except that the albatross of Joe's Alzheimer's is still present.

August 1, 2008—Friday

Joe and I saw a movie with Carolyne and Ed on Friday. Our days have been uneventful. I am still very bald, and am going to wait a couple of weeks before I scare the public.

August 6, 2008—Wednesday

I talked Joe into showering today. He is horny a lot. I think I've figured out why he is hornier after his shower. When he showers and washes his private parts, it feels good, so when he gets out he is ready for a party.

I made him sign a contract, saying that we had completed "dot-dot-dot." In reality, a contract was a waste of time. Joe forgot what the contract said. I guess it was more for me.

August 7, 2008—Thursday

Joe took several naps today, because he kept me up for four hours wanting to *dot-dot-dot* again. I don't think I am going to get him to shower at night. All he thinks about is sex. He continually tells me how much he loves me and wants me. I know all his talk is about what *he* desires. The days of mutual satisfaction are over.

August 8, 2008—Friday

Today, Mindy and I saw Howard, the Alzheimer's counselor. She told him about Joe coming on to her and how frightened she was. She talked about her fears of men. She was frightened at age six by a VA patient standing at our fence. In Dallas, a man chased her when she was jogging. It turned out he was a rapist. He was caught later and jailed. When Joe was JP, we had a lot of undercover policemen dropping by our house for search warrants. I had no idea Mindy was afraid of the undercover police.

August 9, 2008—Saturday

We went out for dinner. I asked Joe what he wanted. He told me to order for him. This is another sign of Alzheimer's. I asked him again, and he said pizza. I told him we had pizza last night, but I should have known that wouldn't matter to Joe. He doesn't remember what he ate thirty minutes ago.

P.S. Joe talks about sex all the time, and tells me how much he loves me. Joe must think he is twenty and a stud. Help!

August 10, 2008—Sunday

Joe showered this morning. I think showering in the morning will eliminate Joe wanting to have sex. I hope so. He has always been sexual. I guess I thought at our age he would slow down, but he hasn't. I miss the intimacy and being with Joe in that way.

Today I worked at the computer, writing in this journal. Because of my surgery, I am now able to type effortlessly.

August 11, 2008—Monday

I have been tired all day. Joe talked and asked questions until 2a.m. He couldn't figure out when we were married. He asked if Thadd and Roy, his deceased brothers, owned this house.

Joe is beginning to worry about his memory loss. Today he told me he didn't want to live his life not remembering our life together and his children. I assured him I would always be by his side to help him remember.

Joe worries that I might give other men attention. I would hate for him to think I would be unfaithful after all the blissful years we have shared.

August 12, 2008—Tuesday

We were running errands today and Joe complemented me on knowing where to go. He said he didn't know anything anymore. I told him I couldn't play the trumpet, so we were even.

After dinner, Joe practiced his trumpet. I told him we were going to play a new game. I would call out a tune and he would play it. He knew every tune I called out. His musical memory is very much intact.

August 16, 2008—Saturday

The annual band reunion tonight was much different than in previous years. Joe sat on the band stand, but never got a signal that it was his time to play. He finally left the band stand, and we spent the rest of the evening visiting with different people. Several of the musicians came by asking him to play. Joe has a unique talent. He has been in the spotlight playing with different bands since age fifteen. Joe toured with Art Mooney and Sonny Dunham for over a year.

Many people who attended the reunion tonight came by and told Joe that they had come to hear him play and sing. Earlier, I had e-mailed one of the guys and told him that Joe will not assert himself to play or sing, so he would need to be asked. That never happened. It was a huge disappointment for our family and Joe's friends. I was looking forward to Joe playing and singing.

I fell in love with Joe's music before I ever saw the man. This last reunion would have been a wonderful birthday present for me. We missed Joe's music, but I took Joe and his trumpet home with me. Every day with Joe is a gift.

August 17, 2008—Sunday

Today is my birthday, and I feel like I'm 78 years old on most days. We all met at the Elite Cafe to celebrate. The girls and I did a pole dance outside the restaurant when we were leaving. It made me feel young.

August 24, 2008—Sunday

A normal Sunday. Church and roast for dinner.

August 26, 2008—Tuesday

When it came time to go to bed, Joe wanted to play around again. He quickly figured out that I was not interested in another night of *dot-dot-dot*, but he still wanted to talk. He began to reminiscence about the old Walkers Auditorium and the songs that were sung. He began singing *Around The Clock Blues* and *I'm Falling For You*. It was late when he finally quit talking. I will always remember this night. Sleeping alongside my "Sinatra," tears come easily.

August 28, 2008—Thursday

Joe wanted to talk again when we got in bed tonight. I thought he was after more sex. He told me how much he loved me and how important I am to him. He told me what he prayed for every night. He kept asking me what our address was. He thought we were on Summer Ave. He lived there when he was in high school. I am glad I didn't turn frigid on him, or I wouldn't have the memories of tonight.

August 30, 2008—Saturday

Because of our pole-dancing outside the restaurant on my birthday, Stacy brought me a DVD by Carmen Electra on how to strip. What a compliment to me! My granddaughter doesn't think I'm over the hill. I love the connection we have. Now I have to try out the moves when my knees are better.

September 4, 2008—Thursday

I met Carol Bice for tea. As I was leaving the house, I asked Joe if he knew where I was going. I had left a note on his wrist, but that note had been forgotten by him as soon as I finished putting it on his wrist. I need to get away more.

September 5, 2008—Friday

Sometimes I don't think Joe appreciates what I do for him. Alzheimer's robs him of anything that was done or said minutes ago. I must remember this is not the Joe of yesterday. He was always more appreciative before the disease.

Joe will not admit he has a memory problem. It seems to me that he thinks if he admits it, the memory problem will become worse.

September 7, 2008—Sunday

Today was Communion Sunday, and for the first time in years I was able to take Communion. My tremor is now under control.

September 10, 2008—Wednesday

Recently, we took our schnauzer, Holly, in to be groomed. She had a seizure, and our Vet called to tell us she was having heart failure. The Vet called later and said Holly was worse. With a heavy heart, Joe and I gave permission for her to be put to sleep. Holly never liked going to the groomer. I will always remember her pleading eyes when she was taken from me. Joe and the twins dug Holly's grave next to Lily's in the back flower bed. Joe forgets both Lily and Holly are dead, and at times, he will ask where our dogs are. I can't stop crying. I have a choice of being downtrodden or enjoying what I have today and the love Joe and I share. It takes less energy to enjoy life and be thankful than it does to frown on what you perceive as bad luck. After a moment of sorrow and grief, we are in charge of making our own luck, and Joe is my luck.

September 12. 2008—Friday

Joe misses Holly as I do. I am going to get us two puppies. Joe will enjoy them.

September 13, 2008—Saturday

I found the breeder where we got Holly. I want to get two puppies so they can play together. Joe is not in favor of two, but I am the one that will be taking care of them, and I don't think two will be as much trouble as one alone.

September 16, 2008—Tuesday

We were sitting in the den this evening, and Joe asked where Iva Belle went. He said someone had honked, and she had taken off in the car with the person. He said it wasn't like her to do such a thing. I explained that Iva was dead, and he must have imagined it. When we went to bed, he wanted to know if he had another wife. He was worried that when his other wife came back, it would cause some legal problems. This was one of those times when I cried. Joe is so confused, and even after living together for fifty-seven years, he forgets who I am. I am sad.

October 7, 2008—Tuesday

This morning, Mindy picked us up for our trip to Austin. Our visit with Dr. Morledege went well. He gave me a prescription of Seroquel for Joe. Dr. Morledege thinks Joe's condition may get worse and that this medicine will take the edge off.

Everyone wants to know if Joe shows any violent or verbal tendencies. Our family and friends worry about me, but Joe is the sweetest, most thoughtful guy anywhere. He may hit his fist in his hand when I tell him where to put his clothes, but he has never laid a hand on me. I'm not sure I want to give these pills to Joe.

On the way home, we stopped to see our puppies. They are so cute and tiny with puppy breath. We must name them before picking them up next Thursday.

October 8, 2008—Wednesday

I had to fill Joe's prescription today, and as we were leaving I was not sure I wanted to give him the pills. I don't want to give him anything that might make him different, or slower.

As we were driving, he looked at me and said, "This is my car." I explained to him that everything he and I own is community property. He replied, "But you're not my wife." This was the first time this particular delusion has ever occurred during the day time.

When we stopped at Gary Boyd's to pick up some papers, we ran into a friend. I introduced Joe to her, and Joe immediately asked about her husband by name. Figure that one out.

P.S. After we returned home from our errands, Joe was himself again. I looked at his daytime delusion as a message from God. I am not qualified to make decisions on my own. I had not asked for guidance, so God spoke to me. I gave Joe his first pill tonight at dinner.

October 10, 2008—Friday

Joe has been looking forward to this band job, and the evening went well. Joe enjoyed being with the band, even though after every job he says that he is going to quit.

October 11, 2008—Saturday

Joe forgets that my legs and knees hurt. When I complain, he takes it personally that I am pissed at him. When he gets himself in that mental mode, he says we are headed for a divorce. This is not a new wrinkle for us. Anytime in the past that I have said I'm tired or am hurting, Joe takes it as criticism of him and wonders if we should continue living together. I wonder from what part of his childhood these comments come from?

October 12, 2008—Sunday

Joe is looking for his mother and sister. I asked him at dinner if he sees them in his mind and if that is why he asks about them? He doesn't know how to answer that question.

It is now 7:30 p.m., and Joe just came to the office window and asked where his sister went. He also thought one of our girls had been here at the house. I couldn't bring myself to tell him that no one is here, nor has anyone been here all day.

P.S. We have named our two puppies. The black one is Abby Lane, and the white one is Allison Belle. We get the puppies next Thursday.

October 13, 2008—Monday

Last night was an all-nighter for Joe and me. Tonight, he asked where his mother was, and then he asked me if I ever talked to Juanita Wills who was Iva's best friend. I knew then that he thought I was Iva. When he thinks I am Iva, he treats me as a guest and says things like, "Do you want something to drink?" "Are you comfortable?" "Are you happy?" That passed after I finally got through to him who I was. If I go along with being Iva, Joe will continue his delusion longer.

When we went to bed, I thought he was fine and we would go to sleep, but I was wrong. From about 11:30p.m. when I turned off the TV until 5a.m., Joe was awake. He went to pee about five times. I think it was stress. Finally, at about 5a.m., I went to sleep. When I woke up at 9:30a.m., Joe was in the bathroom, fully dressed. He said he couldn't find me. I told him I would always be here for him. He said, "I can't be by myself, but that is between me and you." He was still confused.

At breakfast, he told me that as long as I am with him, things are going to be fine. Joe will always live at home with me. He is beginning to worry about himself. As gently as I could, I explained to him that he had Alzheimer's disease—that the plaque in the blood vessels of his brain is the same as plaque in the arteries that cause a heart attack. He accepted that, and I assured him that Dr. Morledge would prescribe any new medication as soon as it was available. Joe then went outside to be by himself.

October 16, 2008—Thursday

We picked up our two six-week old puppies. They slept all night without as much as a peep. Their new home is the laundry room, which is a big improvement from the pen they shared with their sibling.

October 18, 2008—Saturday

I had to make Joe get dressed to go to the hospital. He had been up since 3a.m. and was in a lot of pain. The pain had traveled from under his right shoulder blade, down his back, under his arm, and around to the front. We got to the hospital at 6:30 a.m. Joe saw a doctor and had an EKG, x-ray, blood test, and cat-scan done within an hour. Mindy came to the hospital about 10a.m. By 11a.m., we were waiting for a room. I called the boys, and Jim got Dr. Ritchie to see Joe.

Joe has a blood clot in his right lung. Dr. Ritchie said the clot had done some damage, but his lungs were in good health from the years Joe played the trumpet.

Mindy took the dogs' home with her. I spent the night with Joe.

October 19, 2008—Sunday

Mindy arrived at the hospital by 9a.m, and I went home to rest. While Mindy was there, Joe was confused and wanted her to call me. He was irritated. The doctor wanted him to be still and stay in the bed. He was being given a shot of Lovemox in the stomach to start dissolving the blood clot in his right lung. He wanted to get up. We were up from 6a.m. until midnight. Joe was confused, didn't know what was wrong with him, and was fussy. Dena came by. After the nurse gave Joe a sedative and something in the IV, he soon relaxed.

October 22, 2008—Wednesday

Joe was released from the hospital today. He was glad to be home, but was tired and confused. I have made arrangement to have someone here to help care for Joe.

October 24, 2008—Friday

Joe said he had a hole in a tooth. He was at the dentist two weeks ago, so I thought this was his imagination. But I took him to the dentist, and, sure enough, he had lost two fillings. I apologized to Joe for doubting him.

October 27, 2008—Monday

This is our 57th. Anniversary. We are happy at home learning to live with Alzheimer's.

October 31, 2008—Friday

Everywhere I go, Joe wants to go. I am going to encourage him to stay at home with Priscilla and the pups more often.

We voted this morning. Joe doesn't even know who is running for what. I called out the names, and he would choose one.

November 1, 2008—Saturday

Today, Joe kept saying he wanted to go home. He thinks he is in another city and wants to get back to Waco. Some days Joe is himself, then in the next hour he is forgetful again. This disease plays on my mind. Sometimes I think maybe I heard him wrong, and that I am the one with a memory problem.

November 2, 2008—Sunday

Joe still thinks about sex a lot. I got in the shower with him today, and that was great for him, but not for me. I won't do that again.

With this disease, the person is self-centered and needs to be complimented for everything they do. I am Joe's security as long as I am loving, patient, and close by. Tonight, Joe asked me where I lived, and, as usual, I lost it again. I need for Joe to know me. I need his affection and admiration. Tonight I came to a conclusion of why I react in this negative way when he doesn't know who I am. I go right back to my own childhood. I never felt my mother loved me unconditionally, but I have always felt like Joe loves me unconditionally. When he doesn't know who I am, I am out on a limb alone, and the fear of not having his love causes me to act angrily. When I related all of this to Joe, he told me that my mother had talked to him several times, worried that she had failed me along the way. At least I know now she knew my pain. I am going to bury this injured child within me, forget about the hurts, and think of the good times. There were definitely some good times.

November 5, 2008—Wednesday

This morning, Joe began saying he wanted to go home. He thought we were in a hotel in Vegas. He said he wanted to go where he could talk to his friends, so we went to see Ed. We stayed about thirty minutes. It seemed to appease Joe, although he still thought we were in Nevada.

November 6, 2008—Thursday

Joe wanted to write a thank you note to a friend who had brought us a pie. His handwriting was not good, which indicated to me that he is a sick man. Joe has always had beautiful handwriting.

November 10, 2008—Monday

Joe was very confused today. I never know what brings it on. I was sitting in the den tonight watching him, and I asked myself what I would feel like if he was in a home somewhere and I was sitting here alone. I immediately decided that I will keep him with me, even with his confusion and despair. I would be miserable wondering how he is doing in another location. There may perhaps come a time when Joe will live somewhere other than here with me, but it will be on a day when he no longer knows me. I hope that day never comes.

November 19, 2008—Wednesday

Tonight, Joe again started thinking we were in Vegas. He came in here while I was typing and wanted to know where his keys were, because he was going to drive to a casino and do some gambling. He got testy with me, and told me he was going to get rid of me.

November 21, 2008—Friday

Joe got up this morning, not knowing where he was. After breakfast and several cups of coffee, he was still in the same mood. He was ready to get out of the house, so I suggested we go to Starbucks for coffee. Mindy called, and said she would meet us at Starbucks. I welcome anyone who will visit with us and give me a break from answering Joe's questions over and over.

November 22, 2008—Saturday

Hurrah! Joe got up with no memory problem, and our day went well. I wish this happened more often. It gives me a glimpse into what our days would be like without Alzheimer's.

E-mail to Dena and Mindy:

Dear Dena and Mindy,

I am sending you copies of two thank you notes that Joe wrote. This is not to belittle him, but only to let you observe the place in which I see him. I have read that one can tell about a person's physical health by their writing. This is sad.

Donna McMullen brought Banana pudding, and Joe wanted to thank her. Then when Dena brought the array of nuts and chocolates, I asked if he wanted to write her a thank you note, and he did. He wrote a thank you to Mindy for the CD's and the watch. He keeps going back to the gold one. I ask him if you should take the black watch back, and he said he would wear it too. I will get him to write you a thank you.

I will continue to get him to write, not to belittle him, but to see where he is with this disease.

Thank you for all that you do for us and for stopping what you were doing to meet us at Starbucks yesterday. Joe is more himself today. I think the disease is giving him a rest. I would like to order more days like today.

Love,
Mother

November 23, 2008—Sunday

Joe was back in the limbo mood today. He swept and roamed all day long. Days like today are too long. Yesterday was a good day. Today looks as if it will be an Alzheimer's day.

November 27, 2008—Thursday

Eric, our son in law, hosted Thanksgiving at his office. Joe and I got home about 8 p.m., and Barry came by for a visit. Joe went to bed about 9p.m., and Barry and I stayed up and talked. About 10p.m., Joe came in the playroom, and was obviously angry. I wasn't in bed with him, and when he saw Barry and me talking, Joe was furious. He stormed out of the room and said, "Go to hell." Barry left, and I assured him that Joe would be fine. I got in bed and asked Joe if I could turn on the TV. He grumbled something. I turned on the TV, and lay beside him quietly patting him. He was asleep in no time. He woke up during the night feeling for me, patting me, and telling me, "You are all mine."

November 28, 2008—Friday

When Joe got up this morning, he had no memory of last night. I told him what he had done, and his reply was, "That doesn't sound like me."

December 6, 2008—Saturday

Tonight, I told Mindy and Jim I needed to have a break. Mindy picked Joe and I up, and we went out to eat. When we go out to eat or visit with anyone, Joe always sits with me. I feel like right now I need breathing room, and I am not getting much of it. I am in a slump, but will pull out of it. I don't have much of a choice. I need more help from our kids in order to keep my sanity. Somehow we must visit with friends and family more often instead of staying enclosed in our home. The house is beginning to feel like a jail.

December 17, 2008—Wednesday

In this year's Christmas letters to the fourteen grandkids, I wrote the words to the songs we sang to them when they were babies. I have a letter to each of our children with a recorded tape to help them with the tunes. Joe sang, and I attempted to sing as well. Joe didn't like the way he sounded on the first tape, so he kept singing until he was satisfied with the recording.

December 19, 2008—Friday

We were sitting at the bar in the kitchen today, and Joe's and my conversation went like this:

"I don't know who is sorrier—you or me," Joe said. Then Joe informed me that if I was going to live here in this house, then I should do the jobs that wives do. I defended myself, and told him that he didn't mean those hurtful things, and that I was going to ignore him. But he kept talking, "I think you and I have about come to the end of this marriage." He has always said this when things aren't going his way. By bed time, he was telling me how wonderful I was.

December 31, 2008—Wednesday

We tried to stay up to give each other a New Year's kiss, but had to call lights out at 11p.m. We are getting up earlier and going to sleep earlier these days.

Try as I might, I am never prepared when Joe looks at me with that unmistakable stare of distrust. When he begins talking about how he can't trust me or that he wants to move his money to a safe place, I know I am in for hours of sun downing. I take a deep breath and repeat, under my breath, "He isn't the Joe you know, so be calm and don't take his insults and comments personally." These episodes are coming more frequently. I try to show love and patience. Sometimes I succeed, and sometimes I fail.

January 1, 2009—Thursday

Joe has to open cabinet after cabinet to figure out what he is searching for. Sometimes I direct him or tell him the milk is on the bottom shelf, but this makes him angry. He hears "milk," but doesn't hear "bottom shelf." By the time he hears "bottom shelf," he has forgotten he was looking for the milk.

January 6, 2009—Tuesday

E Mail to Dicque:

My girls think I need an antidepressant because I cry at the drop of a hat. Sometimes I feel like I'm drowning in this ocean of Alzheimer's. I hate pills. I am going to see the counselor I saw last year who told me she thought I was coping fine. She said people cry, but that doesn't mean they are depressed. Sadness is not the same as depression. I get so tired of being upbeat and trying to find some way to entertain Joe. He waits for me to make the first move. I never thought I was a loner, but as times goes by I need my alone time.

Dicque emailed me back:

I can barely imagine what you suffer. You have a lot of pressure to keep everyone happy—Joe, the kids, the grandchildren. This is nothing new because you have never put yourself first. You do need some private time, but how can you do that? You can't even have a break when you two go to sleep at night because you stay busy comforting your loved one until he falls asleep. You may leave, but upon your return you find Joe lonesome and confused. Then guilt attacks. So you take a pill. Then what? The situation remains the same. Relief from your pain comes only with the alternative you don't want: to move Joe to a care facility. It is hopeless and sad, and you two never deserved such fate.

Love to you both.

January 9, 2009—Friday

Joe gets bored when I am journaling. He finds something he needs just to get me up from the computer. Most of the time, I get up and we go sit at the bar and have a coke.

January 15, 2009—Thursday

Joe began sun downing after dinner. He acted like the host, asking me if I wanted something to eat or drink. This indicated to me that Joe didn't know who I was. This lasted until bed time. As we got in bed, Joe looked at me as if it was the first time he had seen me tonight. At that time, I was Deane.

January 19, 2009—Monday

I missed my appointment with Dr. Grayson today. He called me to make sure I was okay. His dad had Alzheimer's, so he knows what I am dealing with every waking hour. Dr. Grayson had prescribed Amitriptyline for me to take in the evening. The girls and Carolyne think I need an antidepressant, but I don't. Who wouldn't have tears when you and your mate are coping with Alzheimer's?

Joe hid his wallet again today. I watched him looking for a place to hide it. He went from one side of the sock drawer to the other, and then he went to the bed-side table, and put the wallet under his pillow. Who knows where he put it last? I had told him that it would be up to him to find it. I asked him to repeat his answer, and his words were, "I'm not going to repeat a damn thing that you say."

I went in the computer to open my e-mails, and I recorded our conversation.

Me: We are married. You don't remember marrying me?
Joe: I presume you have the license with you.
Me: I don't need the damn license. Do you want me to leave? Is that what you want? Do you want me to get out of here?
Joe: That is entirely up to you.
Me: No, I need to get away from you. You don't like anything I do, you think I don't belong here, and you ask me where I'm going to sleep.
Joe: Where is the other lady that is claiming to be my wife?
Me: I don't know what you're talking about. That's what is confusing to you? You think you have another wife?
Je: I am virtually positive.
Me: You are positive?
Joe: I said *virtually*.
Me: What is that supposed to mean?
Joe: Someone else is claiming to be my wife.
Me: Have you heard someone else say they're your wife?
Joe (very low voice): Yes, it seems like I have.
Me: What does she look like?
Joe: Apparently she is not here tonight.

Me: Because I'm the only wife you have.

Joe: Well if that turns out to be a factual circumstance, then nobody is hurt. How do I get into these things?

Me: How did you get into what?

Joe: The situation of two women claiming to be my wife.

Me: Who is the other woman?

Joe: I don't know.

Me: When did you last see her?

Joe: It was yesterday or last night—I'm not sure about that either. Anyhow, I'm not going to fool with it. I will be out of here in a flash and let you all hassle with it.

Me: There is no hassle at all. I am the only woman in your life, though maybe you would rather have another woman in your life. I'm the only woman in your life besides your daughters.

Joe: Are either of them here?

Me: No. They are at their own homes.

Long silence. Joe says something under his breath.

Joe: I wonder where I was when all this alleged matrimony was taking place. I don't know what to do. I want to be fair to those making a claim. I don't want to hurt anybody, and I don't want anybody to hurt me.

Me: I don't know what you're talking about.

Joe: You don't know what *matrimony* means?

Me: I don't know who else said they were married to you. It's all in that vivid imagination of yours.

Joe: No.

Me: So you've been married twice?

Joe: I don't know.

Me: What does she look like? Did you hear her say she was your wife?

Joe: I don't know. How do I get into this kind of shit?

Me: Why don't you go brush your teeth and we'll go to bed? Come on, let's go to bed, and tomorrow will be a new day.

Teeth brushed, dogs bedded down, and Joe and I turn in for the night. Finally!

January 21, 2009—Wednesday

After dinner, Alzheimer's appeared again. Joe mumbled, "How did I get in this mess?" I asked him, "What mess?" He said he didn't know where he was or who lives here. He was so confused. This is a mountain I climb every day until he falls asleep. One minute Joe is himself, and the next minute he is lost somewhere in his mind.

February 1, 2009—Sunday

There isn't much to talk about with Joe. I miss the old conversations. This disease isn't about Joe, it isn't about me, it is about *us*. I must put Joe first. Whenever Joe comes out of the Alzheimer's zone, I have my own free time. Maybe not as much time as I want, but if I do it this way, hopefully it will benefit us both. This turned out to be a good day.

February 4, 2009—Wednesday

Joe has been his old self without any sun downing these past couple of days. I try to imagine how he feels when he thinks other people are in the house, when he isn't sure who I am, and when he doesn't remember we are married. I know that dealing with Alzheimer's on a daily basis is as difficult for him as it is for me.

February 13, 2009—Friday

Dear Dr. Grayson,

I started taking the Amitriptyline, and I still had tears appear out of the blue while taking the medication. I soon noticed that I had changed. I changed from being involved to being indifferent. That is not who I am. I quit taking the pills. I was not communicating with Joe. I wanted to crawl up in my own cocoon. Joe noticed my indifference. I am sure in his frame of mind he was troubled by the stranger I had become. I know I am his security blanket, and even though I enjoy my alone time, he needs the real me. I am passionate in most of my endeavors. For me, crying isn't a bad thing. It tells the world I am human and sad.

If a friend or acquaintance gives me a comforting pat, a caring glance, or a hug, I cry. Some people don't show their emotions like I do. Tears are a part of my past and my present, and there will be tears of joy and sadness in my future.

I think Khalil Gibran said it best in his book, A Tear and a Smile*:*

"I would not exchange the sorrows of my heart for the joys of the multitudes.

"And I would not have the tears that sadness makes to flow from my every part turn into laughter. I would that my life remains a tear and a smile.

"A tear to unite me with those of broken hearts, and purify my heart and give me understanding of life's secrets. A smile to be a sign of my joy in existence."

Thank you for caring, for your time, and for your understanding. You and your family have been on this same journey that I am now traveling.

These are my positive thoughts each day:

1. It is no big deal unless I make it a big deal.

2. Joe has Alzheimer's, but that is not who he is.

3. This isn't about Joe. It isn't about me. It's about us.

Lovingly,
Deane Johnson

February 15, 2009—Sunday

When we got in bed tonight, I kissed Joe goodnight. For the first time in 58 years, he told me he didn't love me. He apparently didn't realize how much that statement hurt me. I began to cry. Joe realized something wasn't normal, and he suggested we go in the play room and have a coke, and we did. We came back to bed, and, still in the fog of Alzheimer's, he asked where he had picked me up. I cried again, fearful that Joe would never know who I am.

February 17, 2009—Tuesday

How long is it going to take me to realize that Joe cannot make decisions anymore? How much longer am I going to deny that we have not just a problem, but a big Problem?

Mindy came over in the afternoon, and explained to Joe over and over again that Alzheimer's causes him to have memory lapses. Joe tells us often that he only has a *mild* memory problem.

I hate to say this, but when Joe acts like this, I don't like him. I know I love him, but at the peak of the fog, I feel like he is fooling with my brain. Some days I feel like I am stranded on a raft, alone with no help in sight. Books say this is a family disease, but I disagree. It is not a family disease but a patient-caregiver's disease. Family has a minor part, but Joe and I have the leading roles. How do I hide my stress and stay upbeat and positive?

March 13, 2009—Friday

Looking back over my journal, I realized Joe has not had a long, drawn out sun downing episode for a few days now. I hope the Lexapro will continue to work this well. This, I can handle.

March 14, 2009—Saturday

I thought Joe was doing well, but today I had a reality check. We went out for lunch and Joe could not order for us, much less for himself. To get through a line and get the food to the table was impossible for him. Reality slapped me in the face, and I am never ready to face the truth.

March 22, 2009—Sunday

I know if Joe was aware of his condition while he is in the "A" zone, he would be upset and tell me I shouldn't have to take care of him. I cannot imagine Joe living away from me. I will keep Joe at home until something drastic happens.

March 22, 2009—Sunday

I am saying goodbye to my lover, my soul mate, the one person with whom I share so many memories. My memories are still vivid, but Joe's memories are fading. The only person on earth who was with me when we made those memories is now losing them. Those memories are falling into the abyss of his mind, all soon to be forgotten. I no longer have anyone with whom I can share our intimate memories. Life is not always fair, but it is what it is. I treasure the memories we are making today.

I am sad to a point, but am happy to be the person to take this journey with Joe. What if he had married someone who was not devoted to him? Looking around, I am a lucky woman to be able to spend all these years with the man I love. He still loves back.

March 25, 2009—Wednesday

Joe is playing a job tonight, and I have encouraged him to practice. But with no incentive, he just ignores me. If he has a thought to do something more than repetitive things like sweeping or picking up twigs, the thought is gone in the flash of a moment, and the guy can't remember what he was going to do.

March 26, 2009—Thursday

Carolyne invited me for lunch at her church to hear a chaplain speak about his wife who had died with Alzheimer's. I did okay. The most troubling thing he said—and I knew this, but to say it out loud brings it home—was that Alzheimer's is the only disease where the patients get worse and there is no hope. Joe, the man with whom I have shared so many special moments, no longer has the ability to share any of our memories. He doesn't remember any of our special times. I have already told myself that there may come a time when he looks at me like I'm a stranger.

I cried during the chaplain's talk, but I will survive this and find some joy and happiness along the journey. I must keep Joe close to me for my sake as well as his.

March 27, 2009—Friday

Before we went to bed tonight, I suggested Joe put his wallet in my drawer under my bras. He said, "Now you will know where it is."

March 28, 2009—Saturday

Joe wanted his wallet before we left the house this morning, but it wasn't in my bra drawer. He must have taken it out last night when I left the room, and hid it somewhere else. We looked everywhere, and he finally told me that he shouldn't handle the money anymore. That was a first for him. He has never admitted that he was not capable of taking care of things.

March 29, 2009—Sunday

We woke up early for church. Joe asked me if his shirt and tie matched. He had a hard time tying the Windsor knot.

When we arrived back home after church, Joe took off his suit and came in the kitchen to ask me for help. He said, "I can't do anything anymore. I don't know where my suit, shirt, tie, or shoes go." I told him not to worry, and that I was happy to help him. He then said, "Don't ever leave me."

March 30, 2009—Monday

Melissa, our helper, is like a ray of sunshine. Having her here to talk to Joe frees me up to go to the grocery store alone. She also makes Joe's breakfast and lunch, and does a thousand other things for us that make our days more pleasant.

March 31, 2009—Tuesday

Before we retired for the night, I found Joe's wallet. He had hid it in his white socks drawer. I told him that I would keep it and give it to him in the morning. For a moment, he bristled and told me he would take care of his own money. But the anger passed as soon as it appeared. I hope I can continue to get his wallet each night and put it up before he hides it again.

April 1, 2009—Wednesday

Joe had diarrhea sometime during the night. What is amazing is that he knew where to get clean underwear. Sometimes when he takes a shower, he will ask where his underwear is.

He slept late, and I noticed he had soiled the sheets. When I asked him about it, he said he remembered he had an accident during the night. Two hours later, he had no memory of the accident and told me I loved making up stuff.

April 2, 2009—Thursday

I woke up early and was having a quiet cup of coffee when Joe walked in wearing only his underwear, looking for me as if he were a small child. I finally convinced him to go put his clothes on.

Sue Bigham, our neighbor, is in Providence ICU, and is not expected to live. That will be a blow to Buck, the girls, and to us too. I feel so badly, because I never took Abby and Allison over to see Sue. She had mentioned several times that she hadn't seen our new puppies. My intentions were good, but I always found a reason to go another day. Now there will not be another day. Lesson well learned: Don't put things off, because you may regret it. I will feel bad forever, but it is a lesson we all need to learn early in life.

April 3, 2009—Friday

Sue, our neighbor died this morning. We went over to visit with Buck. As expected, he is having a hard time.

Joe and I went to work out. When we arrived, he said he didn't know that I worked out too, and asked when I had begun exercising. His memory is going fast. Our "together memories" are no more. This is one of the devastating parts of this disease for the family. Fifty-seven years of memories gone from Joe's mind. I must keep these memories vivid for *me*.

P.S. Around 6p.m., Joe wanted to pay his respects to Buck. He had completely forgotten we had been over there this morning. I called Buck, and explained why Joe was coming over again. I then watched Joe walk over. He stopped several times, as if he were trying to remember why he was going next door.

April 5, 2009—Sunday

This afternoon, Joe asked me if I was watching the show on television, and I said yes. He said he didn't like the show and he didn't like me, and then he got up and left the room. I just let it go. About thirty minutes later, he came in and asked if he could bunk with me. He didn't know where he was. He thought another woman was claiming to be his wife. He didn't know who I was, and after an hour of answering his questions he finally went to sleep.

April 7, 2009—Tuesday

We went to Sue's funeral today. At first, Joe said he wasn't going, but then he decided he would go. I had to pick out his clothes for him. I didn't want him to go out mismatched. He may have Alzheimer's, but I am going to make sure he always looks nice—the way he has always looked. Joe is a clothes horse, but he isn't as particular as he once was.

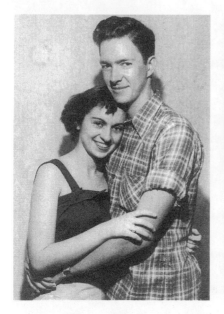 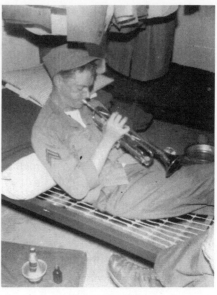

Joe and Deane, May 1951.
Joe's going away party
to the Army.

La Rochell, France. Entreating the
guys in the barracks.

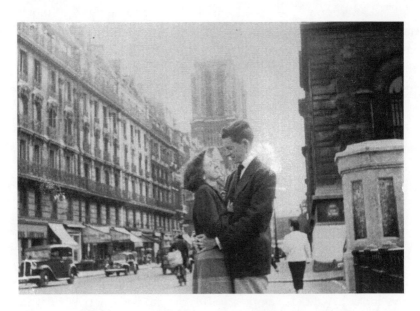

Second honeymoon in Paris, September 1952.

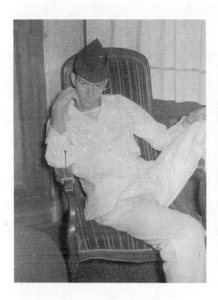

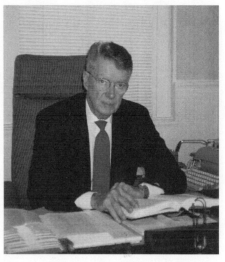

Home in Fouras, France.
May 1953.

McLennan County Court House.
Lawyer and JP.

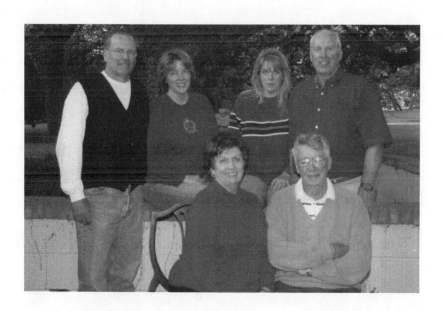

Back Row: Barry, Mindy, Dena, and Jody.
Front Row: Deane and Joe.

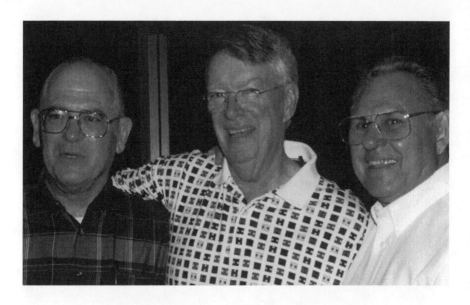

Ed Burleson, Joe, and Nick Klaras. Close friends and fellow musicians.

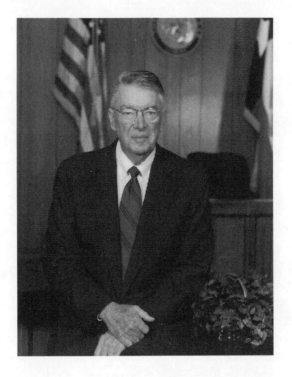

Judge Joe Johnson in court room, 2000.

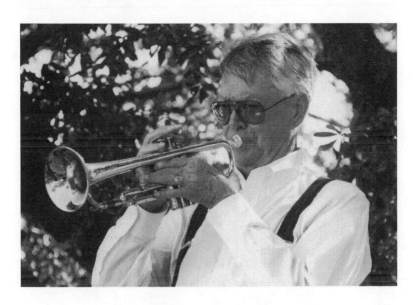

Joe playing outside for 100th Anniversary
of the McLennan County Court House.
September 27, 2002.

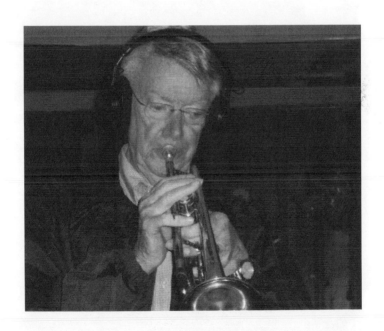

Joe in recording studio, 2002.

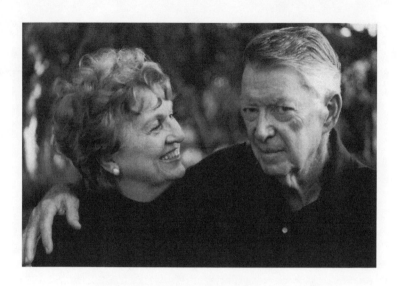

Deane and Joe, 2003.

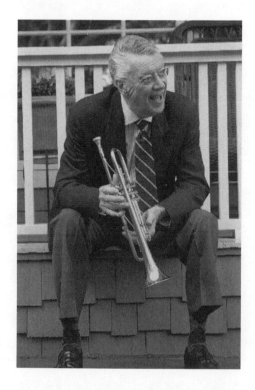

Joe with his trumpet, always laughing.

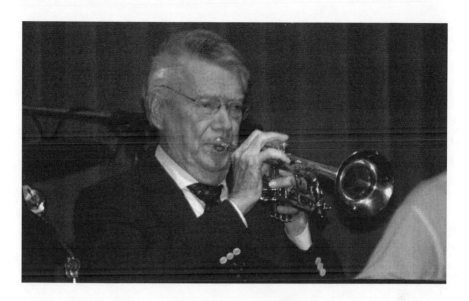

Joe's last job, May 2009.

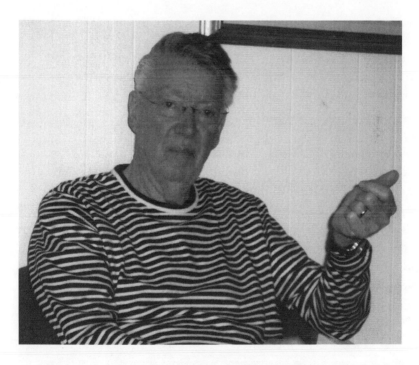

Joe at home, 2009.

April 12, 2009—Easter Sunday

Joe came in the kitchen about 11a.m. In the mornings, he gets up and dresses, but never brushes his teeth or combs his hair. If he doesn't find me quick enough, he fears I may be gone.

Yesterday he followed me into the bathroom. I felt like I was being stalked. I felt his presence while I was checking my e-mail, and I turned and saw him standing in the hallway hiding behind a door. I think he thought I was doing something bad on the computer. Some of the e-mails had audio, and he listened closely, thinking I was watching something X-rated or talking to someone in a chat room.

Before we went to bed, Joe wanted to know who the women were who claimed to be his wife, what our address was, and when we were going home. He kept asking the same questions in bed, and finally drifted off about 11:30p.m.

April 13, 2009—Monday

Melissa couldn't make it this morning, so I left Joe home alone while I went to Dr. Grayson's. I called Joe several times so he would know where I was. During one of the calls, he said, "That is what you told me before you left." I thought, "Good." But he greeted my next call with, "I was wondering where you went."

Tonight, while sitting in the den, he began his questions again. I told him I was his wife and had delivered his four children. He was quiet. I asked if he could name the children, and he couldn't. I named them aloud, and asked if he remembered, and he said, "No." I hate this disease. It is so cruel to rape a person's mind of life's memories. I don't make a big deal when Joe doesn't remember something, even though I am losing my best friend and lover. Joe was the only one around at each child's birth, and he was there the entire time we were raising them. He is leaving me with his empty bag of memories, so it is up to me to remember. I am saddened that I have no one with whom to share these special memories. It seems Joe's most vivid memories are when he was eight to twelve years old. He wants to move back to his childhood home. He thinks if he could move back to Burnett or N. 6th

St., his life could resume the way he remembers. I sometimes wonder how much worse Joe will get, but I don't allow myself to think about it for too long.

April 17, 2009—Friday

This has been quite a day. Joe went with Dena to see the kids' talent show. Dena called me and said Joe thought there was some kind of conspiracy against him. I promptly went to get him. I asked how his dinner was, and he said he hadn't had anything to eat. We stopped at Burger King, and I ordered him a burger. When we returned home, he ate his burger, fries, and another coke. Later, I came to find out he had eaten a chicken fried steak and trimmings earlier.

Within thirty minutes after arriving home, Joe was back to normal—whatever "normal" is. Dena asked me how I deal with Joe all day every day, because, for her, forty-five minutes with him was too much. I asked her if she had ever been in love, and told her I would be with Joe until the end. I can't imagine ever having Joe live apart from me.

April 21, 2009—Tuesday

This is from an e-mail I sent to our children today:

This morning when Joe woke up, he thought I was his mother. It is now 1:30p.m., and I am no longer his mom, but his sister, Iva. He keeps asking me when I am leaving him. I am unsure if he is frightened that I will leave, or if he wants me to leave. Honestly, I feel like it would be a good idea for me to leave, but I would never do that. Do I always respond with a loving tone? No! I am deeply saddened because it is as if all our years together have been forgotten. I know that is the normal progression of this damn disease, but it is heart-breaking and maddening just the same.

Today I am in a valley, angry and sad. If Joe was aware of what is happening to me because of this disease, he would be more concerned and would want to try to remedy the situation. Cancer, diabetes, and heart

problems all have a pill, shot, or chemo to give hope. But there is no hope here. Just a husband and wife meeting this disease together like millions of others. Will I make it? Yes, I will make the best of this badly dealt hand, and will pray daily for a little sunshine along our path.
Love,
Your Mom

April 21, 2009—Tuesday

The day progressed nicely from noon until bed time. At ten 'o clock, we got in bed, and I turned on the TV. Joe asked if I was watching the TV, and I said yes. Fifteen minutes later, he told me to turn it off, now. I should have known that he thought I was someone else, and that he wanted *her* to turn off the TV. I went in the den, and he came in, fully dressed, telling me he wanted me out of the house first thing in the morning. I explained to him that I was his wife. I told him I didn't have the marriage license, but I showed him the hotel receipt from our honeymoon. He was too confused to grasp it. I got up and suggested we go back to bed, but he didn't want me in bed. Finally, we got in bed and he was still adamant about me leaving in the morning. I looked at the clock, and it was 12:48a.m. This session tonight lasted two hours and forty eight minutes. Toward the end, his voice changed, and he reached over and patted me, asking if I was okay. He told me he had had a life-changing experience. He said that when he saw me, he became homesick and lonesome. I brought out the recorder, and for another hour he talked, patted me, and sang.

April 22, 2009—Wednesday

Dena said she had read my e mail, and she asked, "When are you going to find a place for dad to live?" I told her Joe is living with me. I have no intention of ever moving him away from me.

April 23, 2009—Thursday

Jody called saying he had read my e mail. He said he and Barry were busy and could not move back home, but he asked what they could do. I told him if each one of them came for a visit once a month to see their dad, it would be good not only for him, but good for each child to have quality time with him before the disease takes its big toll.

April 27, 2009—Monday

Joe's last long sun downing was April 21st. That is seven days with no sun downing.

May 1, 2009—Friday

Joe's hearing isn't bad, but he has difficulty absorbing the full meaning of a sentence or question. When he says *ugh*, and if I repeat the sentence or question louder, it makes him mad. To him, a loud voice means anger. I can tell Joe to get the coffee cup that is in plain sight, but he doesn't see it—even if he is looking right at it. I wonder if he forgets what he was looking for, or if his eyes truly don't see it.

I am so tired. It has been a long day for me. Joe isn't tired, but why should he be? After dinner, I finally sat down to rest. Joe said he was going for a walk. After twenty minutes, I went out into the front yard to make sure he was coming back. He has only been lost once and that was about a year ago. I opened the front door, and there he sat. He had decided not to walk. I asked him if he wanted to go to Dena's instead, and he was ready to go.

On the way over there he kept talking about being a tease and joker, and reminding me that I belong to him, and that he would never hurt me.

May 2, 2009—Saturday

Joe doesn't know what to do with himself. I am his tour director, and I get tired of being in charge of food, pills, TV program, rides, and conversation. At one time in my life, I thought I wanted to be in control. Be careful what you wish for. I thought after the kids were gone, the grandchildren were older, and Joe was retired, my life would be a breeze, but my days are busier than ever and sometimes I resent it. But I am here for the long haul with Joe by my side.

May 3, 2009—Sunday

Joe and I got up early, and we were ready for church by 9:30a.m. We got to church, and before we ever got in our pew Joe had to go to the bathroom. I stood outside the bathroom door for at least fifteen minutes. I decided right then that we were going home. When we arrived back home, he headed for the bathroom. He doesn't know in time that he needs to potty. I guess by the time his mind knows he has to go, sometimes it is too late.

May 4, 2009—Monday

Joe didn't know how to get his shirt on today. He usually wears shirts that go over his head, and this shirt was buttoned down the front. He couldn't figure out how to get it on or button it. There have been other times when he was trying to put on a coat and couldn't find the top of the coat. The sleeves tend to confuse him, and he sometimes puts the coat on upside down. In the end, I calmly come to his rescue and play it down.

May 6, 2009—Wednesday

Joe has been his old self lately, except at bed time. Almost every night when we get ready for bed, he thinks someone is in the house. It is very real to him.

May 12, 2009—Tuesday

Ed and Carolyne are in Oklahoma, and Ed fell and broke his hip. Luann told us today that Nick is going back to Houston and will be in the hospital for four weeks for some kind of special treatment for his Leukemia. We are all getting old. They may have some hope for their conditions, but we have none.

May 14, 2009—Thursday

When we were in bed tonight, Joe said his mind was messed up. I can't imagine how he copes with this. He really doesn't know what is happening to him. Most of the times he shows no wear or tear, but when he begins asking these off-the-wall questions, I think he knows something isn't right. He just doesn't know what. He has told me that there is a missing link. He says there is a blank spot. I am at a loss on how to answer him. Recently, he asked if he will die from this disease. Luckily, he is upbeat nearly all the time because he forgets these darker questions.

May 16, 2009—Saturday

I was reading an e-mail from Jody written on March 30, 2009. He was responding to the "Folded Napkin" story. He wrote:

A story about Jesus at the Last Supper.
I never knew the napkin was folded. I would interpret the folded napkin to mean that he never left and is with us every second of every day. Our spirit is basis for the continuation of the spirit. Physics teaches that energy never goes away, it is always present, which means that the energy that is generated by our spirit (that energy that we intuitively sense from animals, people, and even from objects) does not dissipate but will remain always. The point is that we all seem to wait for eternity, but we don't have to wait. It is here right now. We just have to be present to recognize it. By the way, this is one of the reasons that I have some peace with Dad's

condition. His mind is affected, but his spirit is completely intact. You can feel the energy.

Have A Great Day,
Jody

May 17, 2009—Sunday

Joe woke up about 7a.m., and immediately began looking for his clothes. He said, "I have to find my car. I need Deane to come get me. I must be crazy. Or maybe I'm delusional!" He then said he should see a doctor. I told him he has been taking medicine for his condition for six years. He said, "Apparently it isn't working." I told him this is the way Alzheimer's affects people. I have been telling the kids that they need to spend more time with Joe, and the time spent with him will be good for them in the long run.

Last night's dinner with everyone, and having Jody here today, has opened my eyes to reality. I figured out that I need the kids more than Joe does. It is a good break from the humdrum days of our routine. Being with them lifts my spirit and gives me something to look forward to. Oh, I look forward to every day with Joe, but honestly I get tired and worn out being the leader, having to constantly be upbeat to keep Joe happy. If I am quiet, he thinks I am mad and unhappy and he reacts to that and not always in a positive way. No one has any idea what it is like to live 24/7 with an Alzheimer's loved one. We are together, but I am alone. I am lonely and lonesome for Joe. I need Joe, and he isn't here for me, not like he once was. Daily help is a must for me, but nothing is better than our children being with us from time to time. Our roles have changed. Joe at one time was my security. But now, having our children on this journey with me is my security. I know that must be a burden for them, but life gave us all a bag of lemons when it gave Joe this disease.

May 18, 2009—Monday

I got up with energy today. Could Jody's visit and all of us going out to dinner have affected me this much? Yes, and I think just having family with us for an afternoon made a big difference.

May 20, 2009—Wednesday

After Joe's shower today, he put on his shorts and then began trying to step into the neck of his t-shirt. He said he was never going to bathe again. I think just getting a towel, stepping in the shower, and shampooing his hair is so frustrating for him. This is second nature to all of us, but he has to remember what to do in sequence and that is confusing.

Tonight in bed, Joe said he was scared. He was afraid someone might come in the house just the same as we do. I explained to him four times about our security system. The explanation went in one ear and out the other. This lasted until almost midnight.

May 23, 2009—Saturday

Our calm day has been rewarding. Mindy and I drove Joe to his band job at the Shrine. The job went great. Joe played for three and half hours without complaining about his lip. During the last set, the band played country western music. Joe just held his horn, refusing to play. When they finally quit playing country western and played what Joe likes, he played.

After Joe plays a job, he gets horny. I guess that goes back to his early days. After a band job, Joe thought an intimate party should follow, and it usually did.

May 24, 2009—Sunday

It was almost 4a.m. before we got to sleep last night after Joe's job. He wanted to seduce me, but I put him off. You may ask why. If we make love, he forgets about it thirty minutes later. The nights of being seduced and making love are over.

May 27, 2009—Wednesday

By the time we went to bed, Joe was in the zone. This lasted about three hours. I can't help but get upset. One reason I do is that many of the things he says take me back to my relationship with my mother. My mother repeatedly told me that she loved me, but I don't think she liked me. She never liked her sister Oleatha, and one day she told me that I was just like her sister Oleatha. I am 78 and should have enough self-esteem by now, but my mother was distant, and now when Joe is distant, my thoughts are, "Why have I wasted my life with these two people who make me feel this way?" I know that is crazy, but when Joe is in the zone, I feel unloved, alone, and in despair. Then, like a curtain going up, Joe comes out of the zone. I am on a rollercoaster ride on these zone nights. In the end, Joe tells me how much he loves me and that our love has been strong from the beginning. Just saying these words erases my loneliness.

May 29, 2009—Friday

Joe was in the zone this morning at breakfast, and I recorded our conversation. He was in his Judge role. He thought I should get an Attorney to make sure no one from my side of the family would claim that I owed them money from what I inherited. I tried to reason with him, but I should know that logic and reason don't work. When I told him that if he was worried, then he should hire a lawyer to look into it and that he would be the one to pay the lawyer, he finally quit trying to make his point. Afterwards, we listened to the recorded conversation. While listening to our conversation, he came out of the zone and said he thought I knew how to handle any situation. One minute he is in the zone, and in the next breath he is out of the zone.

May 30, 2009—Saturday

An e-mail to our children and Dicque:

Life isn't about waiting for the storm to pass; it's about learning to dance in the rain.
Find peace from within. Find love sitting next to you.
Find comfort in the Lord. Find quiet in your heart.
Find me here, praying for each of you.
Love, Mother

Here's hoping June will bring you love, patience, acceptance, and knowledge.

June 2, 2009—Tuesday

Last night was one of Joe's worst nights of sun downing he has ever had. We had dinner, and he was okay. We sat on the back patio with the dogs and then went on the front porch. Joe began asking me where I lived, and I had to get up and walk down the street to keep my cool. He didn't know who I was, and I have not been able to let it slide off my back. I let emotion rule, and that is not good for me or for him. A neighbor stopped and talked to me for a while. I cannot stand sympathy, so a flood of tears began to fall.

We went to bed, and Joe still didn't know who I was. He said he wanted me out of the house and that if I didn't leave he was going to call the police. I tried to calm him, but he wanted me out. I called Mindy at about 10:30p.m., and it took another hour or more to get him out of the Al zone. He wanted Mindy to take me home with her. That sounded great to me, but I can't leave him alone. Mindy managed to get him to take an anxiety medication called Lorazepan (Ativan) that Dr. Morledge prescribed back in March. This is the first time I thought he needed something strong. Sometimes I ask myself how much more I can take. When and if I come to the end of the road, then what?

June 3, 2009—Wednesday

Dena and her boys dropped by. The boys' loud voices and their roughhousing upset Joe. At the time, Dena was telling me about remodeling their house. Joe stood up and went in the house. No one realizes that when they are telling about all they have to do, Joe only hears the anxiety in their voices. I finally told Dena I had to go see what her dad was doing. I don't know if the children and grandchildren will ever understand that my first priority now is Joe. I wish I could still help out or keep a child overnight, but Joe's condition prohibits me from having that freedom. I wish things were different for the sake of my sanity.

Joe was upset almost until bedtime from all the commotion from this afternoon.

June 7, 2009—Sunday

Joe's world is music. He is music. In his mind, he lives back in the 1950's when his band played several times a week. Nightly, he says he is going back to the "old Waco," which are his youth and glory days of music. I think I fit somewhere in his old Waco, but not in his youth and that is where he goes when he is sun downing or restless.

June 10, 2009—Wednesday

Joe began sun downing by 6:30p.m. He said a girl came to our door dressed in a trench coat. He wanted to go look for her. He was afraid she was lost or would get hurt walking in the street. We rode around for a while looking for her just to appease Joe, then we went to Mindy's. I thought if I could get him out of the house and have a change of scenery he would get back to reality. He didn't want to stay at Mindy's, because he was worried about this girl. The scenario of this girl coming to our door was stuck in his mind. For the first time, Jim observed Joe in the Al zone. When we went to bed, Joe was still talking about the girl, and I assured him we would check it out in the morning.

As we were falling asleep, Joe began to sing "It Had to be You," and started a little sex play. Sex is a big part of a man's life, and men often think their sexuality is who they are. Their identity and sexuality, to some degree, are one and the same. We females know who we are without being sexual. Finally at about 2a.m., Joe went to sleep.

June 11, 2009—Thursday

At breakfast, Joe was still sure the girl had come to our door last night. He told me that before Jerry died, Jerry had told him a girl in Mt. Calm wanted to meet him. Jerry has been dead for thirty-five years. When I asked Joe the age of this girl, he guessed her to be about twenty-eight to thirty-five. I told him that the girl would have been a baby when Jerry died. That didn't matter to Joe. Using logic with an Alzheimer's patient doesn't work.

June 16, 2009—Tuesday

We went to visit the Burleson's tonight. Joe asked Carolyne who she was married to. She introduced him to Ed, her husband, Joe's musician buddy for sixty years. On the way home, Joe said he didn't know why he had asked her that question. I assured him no one was hurt.

June 22, 2009—Monday

This evening, I had to make myself dwell on the reality of our present lives instead of what our days would be like without old "Al." Otherwise, I would face disappointment around every corner. I must live in the present, and not think about what might have been. I often find myself thinking of trips we would have taken, conversations about current events, and more time with our kids and grandchildren. I can only dream, but I know most dreams don't come true. That is not my life now, and we will never do those things. I will love Joe as he is and enjoy our days whatever they may be. God will hold my hand throughout this journey.

June 29, 2009—Monday

Today, I told Joe we should brush our teeth in the morning and at bed time. He told me not to lecture him. I wanted to say, "Just let your teeth fall out, ass hole," but I didn't. I just wrote it in my journal instead. I have begun to think more about what our future holds. I looked at Joe, and thanked God for teaching me how to enjoy every moment, because this moment is all any of us have.

July 2, 2009—Thursday

Joe was slower than usual this morning and he has been lost most of the day. After dinner we sat on the front porch, and he asked me more off-the-wall questions like, "Who are you?" and "Where do you live?" I brought out the recorder to let him listen to a recording I had made several weeks ago when he was in the zone. I think our voices on the recording threw him into a ditch. I kept telling him I am his wife, but he didn't believe me. We looked at wedding pictures, and that didn't convince him either. He wanted to take me somewhere, and kept asking where I wanted to go. "We can't live together," he said. I think the mass confusion came from listening to the recordings that I made weeks ago when he was in this same kind of zone. I didn't know how to calm him. He didn't want any part of us going to bed together. He asked me if I had a knife. I didn't, but I wondered if he had gone to the kitchen to get one, and I asked him if he had a knife. "NO," he said. I wasn't scared, but wanted to be sure. I can only try to imagine how he must feel. Here is this strange person telling him stories about his past, and he believes they are lies.

I called Mindy, and Jim answered and said he would come over. Joe wanted us to wait on the front porch for my ride to pick me up and get me out of the house. Jim finally showed up, and, after a while, we all went in the house to get something to drink. Mindy came by and the four of us sat and talked until midnight. I did manage to get Joe to take his nighttime pills about 11p.m., and added the Lorazepan (Ativan) to the dosage. This is only the third time that I thought Joe's anxiety called for a Lorazepan. Mindy and Jim left, and Joe and I went to bed. After we got in bed, Joe kept assuring me that he would never hurt me. I don't think he would either, but, when he is in the zone...? After every sun downing session, he is always so kind, loving, and reassuring to me. Even though he doesn't remember what happened or what was said, it is as if he wants to be the Joe that he really is.

From the book, *36 Hour Day* (page 223):

This is not a problem of memory, she had not forgotten her husband; in fact she remembered him quite well, but her brain could not figure out who he was from what her eyes saw.

I need to remember this when Joe looks straight at me but doesn't know me, or when he wants me out of the house.

July 9, 2009—Thursday

Dear Dr. Morledge,

My journaling shows me that I am now facing reality. Joe does have Alzheimer's. If he has sun downing for an hour or two that means we have an average of twelve to fifteen hours each day during which Joe is alert and aware. I am building my daily life on Faith and Love.

Joe is not always able to figure out how to make a cup of coffee, or a sandwich. He resists bathing and shaving. Some evenings he doesn't know me. It has taken a lot of discipline for me not to react when he doesn't know me. In the beginning, I took it personally. Now, it still hurts, but I have learned to be patient.

As you know, this is a difficult, hurtful, and perpetual disease. I pray, I cry, I get angry, and I journal about our days. Joe is a loving, caring man, and I am forever thankful that I am his wife and, yes, thankful it is me on this journey with him. I do make sure we make good memories every day for my memory diary.

Love,
Deane Johnson

July 11, 2009—Saturday

When Joe is on the phone, he is talkative and upbeat. Then when he hangs up, it is Joe with Alzheimer's. In dark times, the gift of memory and hope sustain us, and give us strength to stand in the face of cruel injustice. Alzheimer's is a cruel injustice.

July 18, 2009—Saturday

Friends ask me if I am ever scared. No, I am not scared, but I am cautious. For example, I don't argue or try to reason with Joe when he is mentally somewhere else. I know that the Joe I know and have been with for almost fifty-eight years loves me. He assures me of this every day. The Joe I know is sensible, loving, and very level-headed. The Joe with Alzheimer's is confused and constantly feels threatened because he doesn't know who I am or where I am. My choice is to deal with the new Joe, the Alzheimer's Joe, the same I would deal with the real Joe—with love and tenderness.

July 23, 2009—Thursday

After Joe showered, he asked where the hair dryer was. I answered, and he said, "Ugh," so I raised my voice. He told me if I spoke that loud again, he was going to hit me. Joe is the baby of the family, and even at age eighty, he feels that no one should speak loudly or harshly to him. My question to him was, "Should I speak louder, or just ignore you?" He replied, "Just ignore me."

July 25, 2009—Saturday

"Is this all there is?" I have to keep putting such thoughts out of my mind. I know that Joe and I have lots of good, loving times ahead. I refuse to allow myself to dwell on this one hour. One bad hour out of twenty-four is nothing. When something bad or disturbing happens to you or a loved one, take care of the problem, and find happiness in the togetherness you share.

July 26, 2009—Sunday

When we were ready to go to bed tonight, Joe asked where I was going to sleep. For the first time, I felt true anger toward Joe for having Alzheimer's. Realistically, I know he would have chosen not to have the disease, but that is not a choice anyone has. I kept thinking, "Joe, how could you do this to me?" I am learning how to cope minute by minute. I must learn how to cope, because Joe is such a sweet, loving guy even when he is sun downing.

July 27, 2009—Monday

I went to the Alzheimer's counselor today. My sessions are always full of tears. Every time, I tell myself I'm never going back, because I don't think I benefit from crying for an hour. The counselor said that when the tangles hit Joe's nervous system the fetal position will show up. I told the counselor I could not picture Joe in a fetal position. My choice is not to dwell on what might happen, but to enjoy the lucid moments and praise the Lord.

July 29, 2009—Wednesday

Joe is worried because he doesn't have any band jobs coming up. He thinks he should go to LA, Vegas, or New York to play his trumpet. The musician in him is the most prevalent of his personality, even more so than his legal career. He worries every day because the music business has gone to pot.

He has developed a tick with this Alzheimer's. If he had it before, I don't remember. Mindy and I first noticed it last October when Joe was in the hospital with his blood clot. He moves his right toe constantly. As he rubs it on the sheet, he makes a swishing noise, and then he pats himself on the back with his hand and makes a slapping noise. I lay in the bed with the knowledge that tonight is more of the same. Would I like to scream? Yes. But what good would it do? How would my life be without Joe? I would rather have Joe with

Alzheimer's than no Joe at all. Joe is living and sleeping with me until one of us passes.

P.S. Mindy and Jim returned home today. I feel more secure knowing she is in town.

August 1, 2009—Saturday

Joe is suspicious of his pill at times. I get tired of explaining what every pill is for. When he gets pissed, I get pissed. Today, he said he didn't want to marry me. I said, "Good. I don't want to marry you either."

A short e-mail from my cousin, Dicque:

I feel for you, and I also feel for Joe. I heard a Pink Floyd song last night with the line, "There's someone in my head, but it's not me," and I thought of Joe. I guess you are grateful that he doesn't know he is drifting away. That would be even more tragic for him if he knew what was happening, wouldn't it?

There is a line from an old black and white movie I saw that made me think of you as you shift back and forth from pretend to reality. It was, "I don't know if I am alive and dreaming, or dead and remembering."

Love you for your patience and courage. How deep is the well it comes from?

Dicque

August 2, 2009—Monday

When Joe got in bed tonight, he wasn't sure who I was, but he said he felt very close to me. He finally quit talking and began singing to me. He sang *Tenderly, Stardust, Cottage For Sale, I'll be Seeing You,* and *I Thought About You.* What more could any woman ask for?

August 3, 2009—Tuesday

Tonight after we got in bed, Joe told me that he doesn't think we should get married right away. Even under these living conditions, there is always laughter if we look for it. Joe has a great sense of humor. He is a funny, happy man—even with Alzheimer's.

August 4, 2009—Wednesday

When Joe was getting undressed this evening, he didn't know where to put his dirty clothes. I know I shouldn't say things like, "Joe you have lived in this house for forty-two years, and the clothes hamper hasn't been moved." I know these words are demeaning. Joe doesn't deserve to be treated this way. He told me he had not lived in this house for forty-two years. I told him we would work it out in the morning, and it seemed like he turned right back into normal Joe again. He spent the next thirty minutes giving me kisses, patting me, and telling me never to leave him. I will never leave Joe. My life would add up to nothing without him.

P.S. Jody called today. Every call from family is a gift.

August 7, 2009—Friday

So what if I get tired of answering his questions? So what if he isn't sure who I am? So what if he doesn't remember where his clothes are? So what if he can't fix himself a cup of coffee? I should and will be thankful that I am the one to be with him throughout this journey. I love Joe more now than I ever have. The life I have with him, even now, is a partnership made in Heaven.

August 11, 2009—Tuesday

When I have help here to interact with Joe, my days are less stressful. I don't mean to imply that being with Joe is stressful, but at times it is. The stress comes when I have to repeatedly answer the same questions over and over. Joe wants to know what is going on with the neighbors, family, and the house. That is to be expected, but because he doesn't remember our conversations, I have to answer him over and over. It gets tiring and stressful.

Buck, our neighbor of forty-two years, is moving. His wife, Sue, died four months ago, and he is selling the house. Sue had been sick for the past five years. When I stand at the kitchen window, I look into their back yard. Sue was a bird-lover. She had wind chimes and bird houses on the porch. There was a magnetic Red Bird in flight on her kitchen window that had been there for years. When Sue was hospitalized for long periods of time, I often looked at their empty house and noticed the Red Bird in the window, the chimes, and the bird house, which all made the house look as if it still had life. Then one day while standing at my kitchen window, the Red Bird was gone. I stood there crying over the absence of the Red Bird, the chimes, and the bird house. I can't talk about the Red Bird without crying. I asked Buck to put the Red Bird back in the window.

I asked Howard, the Alzheimer's counselor, why I am so upset about the Red Bird, the chimes, and the bird houses. He said that I am dealing with loss every day. I see Joe slipping away bit by bit and there is nothing I can do but love what is left. He said that when I saw that the Red Bird was gone from the window where it has always been, my reaction was only natural. I am faced with the reality that ol' "Al" is a permanent intruder. Before Buck moved away, Buck brought me that Red Bird to put on my kitchen window. I asked him about the little white bird house. I told him that I had to face the slow loss of Joe every day, and that now I had to adjust to Buck's departure and the empty window next door—the window where there was once a Red Bird. I can't talk about this without breaking down. The Red Bird in the window was a symbol that nothing had changed, but I know that change is inevitable.

Later that day, I went out on our front porch, and Buck had left the white round bird house for me as well. I have the bird house hanging outside and the Red Bird on my kitchen window. I find comfort knowing that Buck brought them to me to comfort my loss. It is difficult for him to move out of his house of sixty years. He has a new wife now, and a new life. The Red Bird on my window will comfort me every day. It will remind me that life goes on, there is change around every corner, and when friends feel your pain they want to help. The Red Bird on my kitchen window is mine. This little Red Bird reminds me there is life and joy in each day.

August 12, 2009—Wednesday

Joe slept until noon. Howard said Joe would be less likely to sun down if he was rested. I told him that Joe seemed to be tired even when he slept a lot. Howard said the brain is overworked with Alzheimer's. The person with AD trying to do the little daily things gets tired easily. An overworked brain is an overworked Joe.

August 14, 2009—Friday

Tonight, I lay in bed wishing we could recapture our lustful love. I wished for a conversation about a current event. I wished for just one more visit with Joe before Alzheimer's. If the day comes when I am a stranger to Joe 24/7, I hope his heart remembers that I love him and he feels safe knowing I love him.

August 15, 2009—Saturday

Joe slept late. I had a lot of quiet time this morning. We made up the bed together. Joe can't remember where the pillows go. Before ol' "Al" made tangles in Joe's brain, Joe used to make up the bed and knew exactly where every pillow went. It is obvious that Joe can't make decisions about much of anything anymore. This disease does to the brain what ALS does to the muscles.

August 17, 2009—Monday

I cried this morning, because Joe didn't remember that it's my 79th Birthday. He *can't* remember. I am sad, not because he doesn't remember. I am sad because I am alone even with Joe by my side.

As we were lying in bed going to sleep tonight, I missed Joe telling me, "Happy Birthday girl." In all years past, before we went to sleep, he would tell me that he wished me many more birthdays and that he hoped he would be around to celebrate with me. It is these kinds of little things that make this journey with Alzheimer's so trying, constantly sad, and lonely.

August 18, 2009—Tuesday

At times, I don't like Joe. *Is this what my life is going to be like, day in and day out?* I wonder.

I am thankful that I don't harbor these feelings for long periods of time. I insult Joe when I question his lack of ability to explain. When he says he doesn't remember something, I will often say something like, "That doesn't surprise me." I want to leave and not come back to the Alzheimer's. I don't want to do this anymore. I want to get rid of the underlying love I have for Joe, then I wouldn't feel so guilty when I am an ass hole to him. I want our life back. My disappointment, my stress, my anxiety, my tiredness, my anger, my lack of patience, my selfishness, portrays a vision of me that I am not proud of. I am ashamed to be this weak and unloving. How am I supposed to cope and love him with all my heart, but not forget myself while I am living this life every day? I can answer my own question. To love and enjoy all our days, I have to accept the shortcomings, the sun downing, and live one day at a time. Always live in the NOW.

P.S. Joe is looking for his trumpets. He has four trumpets, and he can't find his mouth piece. He had his mouth pieces out a few days ago, and I cautioned him not to hide them like he does his wallet. I got up and luckily I found the mouth piece in his top drawer. He made a joke about hiding things and then began to make up a song. I wish I found it funny, but I don't.

Later, we were almost asleep, and Joe whispered in a quiet voice, "Who is in bed with us?" I wonder if this is another stage, a onetime only question, or just another piece of the Alzheimer's puzzle?

August 26, 2009—Wednesday

After three hours of sun downing, we went to bed at 7:30p.m. Joe woke up an hour later and thought we were in a hotel. He put on his clothes and began looking for an elevator. I kept trying to get him to come back to bed and go to sleep, but his mind was racing. His next thoughts were that we were in a flood and needed to take cover. About 3:00a.m., I got up and went to another bed. I was almost at the end of my bag of tricks. When I got in the other bed, I heard Joe getting up and saw the hall lights go on. I warned him not to open the outside doors, because the security system was on. His worries suddenly changed. Joe wanted to call the police to go to Cameron Park and make sure our kids were safe. In his mind our children were in danger of drowning in Cameron Park. I decided to turn off the security system, and we sat on the front porch. My hope was that if he saw we were at home, it would break the "Al" zone. But he took off down the street looking for a police car. I insisted he come back, and he eventually did. I told him we had to go in the house because if our neighbors saw us sitting on the front porch at 4a.m., they would call the police. These discussions lasted until 5a.m., and he finally wore himself out and went to sleep. I got four hours of sleep before I had to wake up. This was Joe's longest sun downing. It was stressful for me, but I can't imagine how distraught he must feel worrying about our kids. I wish I could help him understand that none of these thought are real, but I can't. What do I do?

August 30, 2009—Sunday

An Email to our Kids:

Dear Jody, Barry, Mindy, and Dena,

I am sending some pages from my journal. I need for each of you to know what my days and nights are like. I am honest in my writing about your dad, about my stress, and about negative feelings dealing with this disease on a daily basis. Every day I put it all on paper and then try to find a way to deal with the ups and downs of the disease.

When reading, I hope you understand the anger I express at times and that you don't feel bad toward me. I love your dad and want to be the best I can be as a wife and caregiver. But this is a lonely journey.

I know you all have families, and I don't expect you to drop everything and come to my rescue. Jody and Barry, I know you can't come in a moment's notice, but I may need to call you and have you call back to talk with your dad sometimes. It may help him break out of the "Al" zone. Last Wednesday night I fooled with him from 9:30p.m. until 5a.m. Boy, did I need help. We were sitting on the front porch at 4a.m. Mindy, I have called on you and Jim so often I don't want to work a good horse to death. I would never bother any of you for something insignificant. I have tried not to impose on you and will not impose in the future unless I am at the end of my bag of tricks. The books say this is a family disease, but I beg to differ. I find Alzheimer's disease to be the Alzheimer's patient's and caregiver's disease. As I said above, this is a lonely journey.

I pray that Joe doesn't get a lot worse, although he began sun downing before noon today. Mindy picked him up to take him out to dinner, and he asked me, "Is this the end for you and me?" He was worried that I wouldn't be around when he got home. You have all urged me to get help, and I have and will probably have more in the near future, but I can't predict when the sun downing will begin or how long it will last. It would be foolish to hire someone 24/7 at this time. No, I am not putting your dad in a home. This I can manage, but I might need to call every once in a while for backup.

I urge you to visit when you can, call and talk to Joe often, and know that I love you. At one time, Joe and I were your security. Now, you are our security. I am Joe's sole security, and that is quite a job and all the while a rewarding one.

Lovingly,
Mom

September 2, 2009—Wednesday

An e mail from Dena:

Dear Mom,

I want you to know I love you and Dad very much. You are a strong woman and sometimes it takes tremendous strength to do very difficult things. I need you to know that I am a phone call away. My first responsibility is to my family—Eric and the boys.

If you need me and I can help, I will. If I can't, for whatever reason, I will tell you.

I will not participate in your refusal to get help for yourself and Dad. I have some idea of what you deal with, but of course cannot fully know the *extent of your struggle with Dad's illness.*

I want to encourage you to please get help from people who are qualified to give you and Dad the professional help you need and deserve.

I am a phone call away and I love you very much,
> *Dena*

September 5, 2009—Saturday

I read Dena's e mail, and I know our children have concerns about me. I cannot bring myself to allow Joe to live apart from me. I just can't.

Joe and I went out for dinner tonight. He went to the restroom, but couldn't find the exit door to get out. When another man went in, Joe then figured out how to exit. When he got back to the booth, he told me he didn't know how to get out of the restroom. He didn't seem upset, but I know he must have been when he stood in the restroom with no idea how to get out.

September 9, 2009—Wednesday

E mail from Dicque:

After reading the small part of your journal, I'm convinced you could make your own movie.

I was happy to learn from your journal that Joe still has moments of clarity when you two sit together and talk. But what gets me are those shocking spells of panic when his memory fails him and he "disappears" from you. You might think that your reactions to him are sometimes cruel. That's understandable. You'd think you'd get used to his spells, but I'm sure it comes as a shock each time! I don't know how you cope as well as you do.

Your journal made me feel as if I were spending each day with you.
> *Love,*
> *Dicque*

September 25, 2009—Friday

Jody called today, and talked to Joe while Joe was fully sun downing. Joe said he wanted to go back home, and that he and Iva could not get along (referring to me). He asked for Jody's phone number in case he needed him. The conversation lasted at least thirty minutes. In the end, Joe made the comment that he wasn't going to hurt anyone. I got on the phone to assure Jody that we were okay. I told Jody that Joe thought he was talking to his brother, Roy, who has been dead for twenty-seven years.

We started to bed at 9:30p.m., and Joe waited to follow me because he didn't know where the bedroom was. Lately, Joe is convinced other people are here with us. He can't give them a name, but he walks down the hall looking for the guys and girls he says he saw here.

When we finally got in bed, Joe told me "I don't want any tonight." I thought that was the best thing I had heard all day.

P.S. I wonder how much of me is left to deal with this disease.

September 27, 2009—Sunday

In my earlier journal entries, I repeated these two quotes many times: 1) It is no big deal unless I make it a big deal. 2) Joe may have Alzheimer's, but that is not who he is.

Now, I have to revise those statements to, "It is a big deal, and at times Alzheimer's is who Joe is." I want my husband back. I want to respond to Joe with affection and love, but that is hard for me at times. I'm sure most people would wonder why. The truth is that the man I live with is Joe, but this Joe with Alzheimer's is unable to share his feelings or even have a conversation about what we did last night. The only conversation he is capable of having is, "I want a kiss." "I enjoyed my lunch." "Where are our dogs?" and "Who are you?" I must learn to live in this new world, this smaller world. I must find joy in this environment in which we now exist.

October 2, 2009—Friday

When we were eating dinner tonight, Joe said, "Honey, you know the girl that was here today, does she have a home somewhere?" He didn't remember Melissa, our helper, even though she is here all day, three days a week, and even some evenings.

Joe sun downed from 7p.m. until midnight. He was really confused. He didn't know who I was, and he didn't remember we had kids or what town he was in. He also was worried about his trumpet and if he had any money.

October 8, 2009—Thursday

Mike Copeland with the News Tribune came by to get the piece I wrote for Joe as a tribute to Nick. Joe staggered into the den, barefoot, shirt all disheveled, hair uncombed, and in need of some personal maintenance. Joe has always been a clothes horse, but now he is always in too big a hurry to find me that he forgets to groom himself. Joe is almost eighty-one, but his actions remind me of a two year old.

I asked Joe how he felt when he was confused. Adamantly, he said that he wasn't confused, but he just couldn't get anything done the way he once could.

October 9, 2009—Friday

Joe was himself all day, but he began to sun down around 8p.m. He didn't know who I was. He refused to get in bed with me because he said other women were claiming to be his wife. After a few hours of this, I stopped being mellow, caring, and loving toward him. I clammed up until Joe finally fell asleep, then I cried myself to sleep.

October 17, 2009—Saturday

Tonight, Joe woke up and said two men were here and up to no good. No one was here except for Joe and me. He was sure the men had set something on fire. Joe wanted to know which of the men he saw sitting in the den had set the fire. Joe was talking to chairs and pillows as if they were people. In his altered mind he saw the men sitting in chairs in the kitchen. He pulled his chair close to the red chairs, and pointed his finger and began telling the men (i.e., chairs) that they had nothing to fear if they would tell him what they were doing here and who had started the fire. Joe said he didn't want to hurt them, but that he wanted them to tell him why they were here. He introduced himself as 'Judge' to the men. Joe was certain he saw two men here sitting in chairs in the kitchen. He wanted me to call the sheriff to come and get the men. Then Joe started walking down the street looking for the two men. He finally came back in the house, but stopped at a full-length mirror in the foyer and began talking to his reflection.

When Joe and I got in bed, he thought we were going to have sex. He got up when he realized nothing was going to happen. He lives in the past when he was once capable of performing nightly. He thinks he is younger. Joe will not allow himself to believe that age has stolen his ability to have sex. He told me that he was paying $45.00 an hour for the room that we were in. If we didn't have sex, we were wasting our money.

I called Mindy, hoping her presence would bring Joe out of the zone. Jim came with her. Joe began telling Mindy and Jim that he was paying for the room by the hour and that the money was wasted if we (Joe and I) didn't use the room for sex. When I showed no interest, Joe felt rejected and got annoyed—not mad, but annoyed. Thankfully, the moment passed, Mindy and Jim went home, and Joe got in bed and went to sleep.

October 18, 2009—Sunday

I gave Joe half a sleeping pill tonight and he went to sleep—or so I thought. He kept talking about one thing, then another. It finally dawned on me about 3a.m. that Joe was not awake. He was sleeping while reciting what he was dreaming at the moment.

The first dream was a car traveling toward us, getting closer and closer. Next we were on a train and the waitress was fixing us a tray of food. Joe was telling about the salad, meat, and dessert. I thought maybe he was hungry. I asked him if he was and if he wanted me to fix him something to eat. He said, "No." His next stop was in Paris, and he was telling about touring the city.

What is happening? This isn't like Joe.

Dena sent an e mail today about a lost dog, titled, "I Found Your Dog Today." This was my response back:

Dena, I didn't need something else to cry about. As I read this I thought of your Dad's eyes, lost, searching. He looks at me and I am that stranger who reached out to pat the dog. I offer my hand, and he turns away. He doesn't see me. Joe is drowning in confusion. I look for Joe and although he is standing right in front of me, I don't see the man of yesterday. Joe stands tall, handsome as ever, yet so far away. Joe is searching, he is scared, and he is asking questions and wanting me to help him understand what is happening to him. I can't help him across this bridge, and he gets upset and frustrated with me. I hope in his heart that he remembers how much I love him.

When the dog died, I hope the comfort from the stranger let him know he wasn't alone. Joe will never be alone. My heart is connected to him now and forever. I feel alone. I pray that Joe finds comfort in all the strangers that invade his mind daily. I wish, I pray, and I, along with Joe, am drowning in fear, loneliness, and sadness.

What a wretched disease Alzheimer's is.

> *Love,*
> *Mom*

October 19, 2009—Monday

Mindy spent the night with us. Joe narrated his dreams for most of last night. He woke up at 5a.m., and said a preacher came in and stole his shoes. He was angry, pacing the floor, looking for the new shoes he said the preacher man had stolen. He walked down the hall hollering, "Preacher!" Mindy and Joe went to McDonald's at 6a.m., hoping that by getting Joe out of the house, Joe would leave the A-zone.

Joe is more often in the zone than out of the zone these past few days. I am baffled. What do I say? What do I ignore? How do I lead him into my world and out of his? His world is a place I want to avoid, and I wish I knew how to lead him out of that miserable place. I pray, I hope, and I cry.

October20, 2009—Tuesday

I called Dr. Stern and told him about Joe's problems. He sent out Divalproex for agitation. I had thrown the Mirtazapine and Lorazepam away even before Dr. Stern told me to. I think I overmedicated Joe and that was the cause of his agitation and delusions these past weeks. The medicine should have calmed him and helped him sleep, but he reacted totally opposite. I was looking for help in the form of a pill, not realizing that the pills were making Joe's condition worse. I wish I had used some common sense, but I was traveling in the wilderness. No more of those pills.

Jody and Barry came in to meet with Howard the Alzheimer's counselor along with Mindy, Dena, and I. We were telling Howard about Joe's confusion the last few days. This gave Howard the impression that it was time to find a home for Joe. We all went to an Alzheimer's facility, and listened to the Administrator. We walked thru the facility, and I was in pure shock. No way was I going to put Joe there. I will have around the clock help in our home forever before I place Joe in a home away from me. I cried and was sick with grief. I was fearful for Joe and myself. I have always known that I am deeply in love with Joe, but while walking through this facility, I began to feel a love for Joe that I had never experienced before. It was an overpowering kind of love. It was kindred to the love a parent calls upon to protect the little ones she loves. It is the deep love that a wife has for her mate. For the first time in fifty-eight years, I loved Joe unconditionally. I was sick, thinking, "How could I have thought of placing Joe anywhere other than with me?"

The girls went home. Jody, Barry, Joe, and I went to Casa for dinner. They were thinking that Joe was going to be evaluated on Wednesday (tomorrow), and that he would be admitted to the facility on Thursday. I knew then that my kids didn't really know me. I was sick at heart. I was as low as I've ever been. I was ready to pack Joe and myself up, and disappear. I know all four kids said it was my decision, but I also knew they thought I should do something. No, I'm not going to be separated from Joe. So what if I am aging? So what if I don't get out daily? So what if my very being is wrapped up in my husband? That is what I want. I want to be wrapped up with Joe forever until the day of departure comes in death. I will welcome that ending as a gift for the two of us. I hope that doesn't sound callous or mean. There are some things worse than death.

October 21, 2009—Wednesday

I got up early to make the necessary arrangements to hire help for Joe and me. I called Visiting Angels to request help in the evenings and on the days Melissa isn't here. I called the Alzheimer's home and canceled Joe's evaluation today. I didn't want to waste any time fixing what needed to be done in order for Joe and me to have as close to a normal life under these circumstances as we possibly can. I will play this by ear. I will have help here every day for me, and be able to love having Joe here with me in our home. There isn't any question in my mind about how I can do this. I will be by Joe's side now and always.

October 22, 2009—Thursday

Jimmy Johnson, our minister, came by for a visit today. I told him that Joe sleeps late, and if I don't get him to shave and shower on Saturday, it is impossible to make it to church on Sunday morning. Jimmy's answer was, "In retirement, one needs to sleep."

October 25, 2009—Sunday

I find myself praying all the time. I am not praying for Joe to be free of AD. I am praying for direction and guidance for me so I can take care of Joe and in some way eliminate or make his sun downing light and short. I am praying our luck holds out until our time on this earth is over.

October 26, 2009—Monday

Dena called, and Joe and I picked up the phone simultaneously. He told Dena he was trying to get our stuff packed up so we could leave. I went to the back, and it was true—he really had emptied my jewelry drawer, all his shaving things, my make-up, and taken the toilet paper off the roll to pack that too. He was in the zone big time.

When we were in bed later, the zone returned. Joe was convinced we were at the Raleigh hotel on the fourth floor. He wanted to call home to have someone come and get us. I kept telling him we were home. He said he would call the police to come after us. I told him to go ahead, but in the long run he would be embarrassed. The police would tell him he was home and later tell their fellow officers about the house call to the Judge's house with comments like "The Judge has lost it." Joe didn't like that.

October 27, 2009—Tuesday

Today is our fifty-eighth wedding anniversary.

I don't know why I get so disgruntled with Joe. I feel like my jobs are multiplying every day. I wonder how much more I can do. Can I accomplish all that needs to be done taking care of Joe and the pups? As always, my needs are last priority. Can I keep my energy level high and my anxieties low in order to do what I expect of myself and what Joe expects of me? No one takes care of me except me. In Joe's mind, he can do anything and everything he has ever done. He will not acknowledge that he has any kind of problem. He doesn't think I have that much to do. He taunts me by saying it doesn't take much effort to make a cup of coffee or a sandwich. Joe's solution is to call our daughters to do my job. I told him they have families and that not one of them is prepared to give up their life to help here. I told him that, after he spent one night with his aging mother, he said we needed to find a nursing home for her, and we did. Of course, she was ninety-five years old. Even so, I must learn to have more patience and quit feeling sorry for myself.

When we got in bed tonight, Joe asked me if someone had set his bond. He thought he was in jail. I assured him we were at home.

Do I have clothes here? he asked.

I paused to think about how I might feel if I didn't know where I was, if I thought I was in jail, not knowing if I was at home, wondering where home was, and not sure if my clothes and car were here in this strange place. What if the stranger beside me kept telling me everything was okay, that I had never been in jail, and that my clothes and car are here? I can hardly imagine what Joe goes through in these moments.

October 28, 2009—Wednesday

Joe's questions are as rapid as a machine gun. If I ignore his questions, I can tell it annoys him.

At midnight, I turned on the light and said to him, "If you're not going to let me sleep, then let's get up." He didn't want to get up. I told him his constant questions were a form of torture to me. We finally got to sleep by 1a.m. I can't go to sleep until I hear his breathing even out, which tells me the torture session is over. I pray for a way to answer Joe's questions to his satisfaction.

October 29, 2009—Thursday

Tonight, I started early in the evening telling Joe where we were, and who I was. We got in bed, and I continued repeating, "We are at home, where we have lived for forty-two years. I am your wife of fifty-eight years, and all is right with the world." We were both happy and calm.

Thank you, God, your prescription worked! Joe had no sun downing, and he went to sleep just like a baby. I went right to sleep too.

October 30, 2009—Friday

Tonight, I continued telling Joe who I was, where we lived, and so on. So far it is working. When we got in bed, he asked a few questions. In a calm, loving voice, I answered, reassuring him that we were in our home. A home he built for us. I complemented him over and over. I praise God for showing me a way to comfort Joe. This is working.

October 31, 2009—Saturday

Joe swept the driveway and patio this afternoon. For Joe, a twig is a call to sweep. I am determined to have him record more albums. I found most of the lyrics to the tunes I have picked out. Joe practiced five or six tunes tonight. I called out a tune, and he played it.

November 10, 2009—Tuesday

Joe woke up this morning and thought he had to go to school. I asked him if he knew how old he was. He thought for a moment, and couldn't come up with an age. He worried about getting to school on time. After explaining to Joe where we were, he began to come out of the zone. He told me he didn't know how he would manage without me. He knows he has Alzheimer's, but he hates the word. He told me I was a good person, and that I never made fun of him. I am happy that Joe feels the love I have for him and knows how much I love him.

The Lord is paving our way. Amazing!!!

November 18, 2009—Wednesday

We were watching TV after dinner, and Joe got annoyed with me. I had used a tone of voice that escalates the zone he is in. I began my monologue, and he told me he didn't believe anything I was saying. I said, "I love you," and he said, "I like you, but I don't love you when you act up." During these exchanges, I had a flashback to my childhood when I would tell my mother that I loved her, and her response would be that she loved me when I was a good girl. The little child in me has not yet healed.

November 19, 2009—Thursday

I met Marceline for lunch. She is a high school friend of mine.

When I got home, Joe was annoyed and wanting to know why I was so late. It is hard to get away from him for a private outing. Joe has no idea how tied down I feel. If I get on the computer, he is asking for me every twenty minutes. I think he would be happy if I sat by his side 24/7.

Sun downing alert: We got in bed, and Joe asked questions for an hour. It is so strange. We were in the bed, he didn't know me, didn't know where he was, and he asked about his mom, his siblings, and where I lived. Then, as if the curtain was raised, he reached over and patted me. He knew who I was again. Twenty minutes ago, he was distant and reserved. Now, he is Joe, saying, "If you need anything in the night, don't hesitate to call me." Sometimes I wonder if I am losing my mind. I ask myself, "Is this for real? Did I imagine that Joe didn't know me? What is going on?"

November 20, 2009—Friday

This evening, Joe began to roam from one room to another. By the time we were going to bed, he didn't have a clue who I was or where he was. He said he wanted me to get out. He said he was going to call the police to come and get me. He asked me if I was drunk, and said, "If you're not drunk, then you must be crazy." This lasted for half an hour. Later, we were in bed, and he had his back to me. He reached over to pat me, and asked me if I was okay. The Alzheimer's veil had been lifted.

November 22, 2009—Sunday

Dear Dr. Morledge,

Last night Joe and I were listening to jazz, and he asked me to dance. We were dancing, and I thought everything was good. But when he sat down, he looked at me and didn't know who I was. He said he wanted me out of the house and that I didn't belong here.

Our kids ask if I am afraid of him. No, I'm not afraid, but when Joe is in the zone I am careful not to say or do anything to offend him. He isn't Joe when he is in the zone. He is a sick man with a despicable, heart-wrenching disease.

I will sum up our days in this way: Joe and I have less than two hours of sun downing each day, we sleep eight or nine hours, and that leaves fourteen hours that are pleasant and close to normal. Someway, somehow, I will find a way for Joe and me to live in our home with love and grace. I am Joe's security.

I continue to write, because writing is one of my outlets. I am getting out more with friends. I am living, knowing my days with Joe are numbered. I will love and relish being Joe's wife until the end.

Lovingly,
Deane Johnson

November 26, 2009—Thursday

Today is Thanksgiving at Eric's office, and I hate to admit that my disposition is rotten. We celebrated Joe's birthday today instead of tomorrow.

November 27, 2009—Friday

At 1:30a.m., Joe put on his clothes, and told me he was going home. I tried to talk him into coming back to bed, but he was deep in the Al zone. He roamed through the house looking to see who was here. He called me to the den, and said a man was trying to push some boys off the bridge.

In the den, I have sixteen-inch statues of two babies playing. Joe had put the statutes on the floor, worried that the "man" was going to push the babies off the bridge. I explained to him that the twin babies were made of plaster. Joe said he knew that, but he could not sort out the delusion from reality. I began pampering him, talking sweetly, telling him I needed him in bed with me. I said, "I can't go to sleep without you." At 3:30a.m., he finally came to bed. When I knew he was asleep, I went to sleep too.

November 28, 2009—Saturday

I was telling Joe about last night, and, of course, he had no memory of the event. He told me I should see a doctor. Joe has always been that way. If something is wrong, it is certainly not his fault. It is always the other person who is wrong or needs help.

We kept talking, and I think he finally understood that he was the one in the zone. He told me again that I shouldn't have to put up with him in that frame of mind. I assured him that as long as I can handle him in the zone, he will stay at home with me. I told him that we should shower tonight, so we can go to church tomorrow. He asked me not to take him anywhere if he would embarrass me or himself.

Recently, I had Joe sign a contract promising that he would practice his horn every day at 2p.m. I explained to him again how important it was for him to use his brain. Today, he practiced for about thirty minutes. Joe's incentive is gone, and it's sad because he plays so well.

Did I really think Joe would remember signing a contract? That was wishful thinking on my part. I guess it is natural to grab at straws.

Later, I lay in bed just thinking. When Joe asks me any question like, "Where do the dogs sleep?" instead of me saying, "They sleep in the laundry room," I answer him in a belittling way like, "They are sleeping in the same place they have slept for a year." When I belittle or demean Joe with an answer to his question, he soon forgets the sarcasm. But I realized that I will feel guilty and ashamed about my unloving, sarcastic answers until the day I die. This realization was a wake-up call to give me peace and free me of guilt today and for all my tomorrows. This was a nudge from God. I will do better.

December 13, 2009—Sunday

Sometimes just the sight of Joe depresses me. If he could change, I know he would. The man I love is sick. He doesn't have diabetes, heart trouble, or cancer. If he did have any of these, we might have some hope. But we have no hope.

December 20, 2009—Sunday

Blake, Jody's oldest, walked throughout the house remembering his visits years ago. Joe enjoyed everything about the day. With all the people around him, he was the old Joe with just a touch of Alzheimer's. I wish he would stay this way.

December 21, 2009—Monday

This morning, we were having breakfast, and Joe asked me what time it was. I told him to look at the clock. He looked at the clock, and didn't even come close to the right time. This was a FIRST!!! I felt like I had been zapped with a stun-gun. I doubt if I will ever fully accept that Joe cannot remember the simplest of things. It is so hard for me to understand.

December 22, 2009—Tuesday

While at the grocery store last week, I began quizzing Joe with the same questions Dr. Morledge had asked him—the questions Joe couldn't answer. But Dr. Moreledge had asked him these questions before Joe began taking the Axona Protein drink. I asked Joe what was the big holiday we celebrate in November, and his answer was Thanksgiving. The next question was, "What holiday is in December?" His answer was Christmas. I didn't think much about it, but then at the symphony on December 11th, he introduced me to a lady that works at the Court House. He didn't know her, but she made herself known to him. He said, "This is my wife, Deane, of 58 years." I was shocked. He hasn't known our anniversary or how long we've been married for years. I wondered if the Axona was already working after only 11 days. But it was probably just wishful thinking.

December 25, 2009—Friday

Christmas note to friends:

Happiness is being close to family and friends. Every day is Christmas, but you may have to look under a rock or two to find Santa. Joe is doing well, our family is healthy, and life is sweet.
Merry Christmas,
Deane and Joe Johnson

December 26, 2009—Saturday

Joe and I went to the movie theater to see *Blind Side*. He talked about the movie until bed time. Is the Axona protein drink working?

Blake called, and so did Jody. I love hearing from the grandchildren. I like knowing they feel connected to us. In this world of Alzheimer's, I need to know I have family in the wings who think of me.

December 27, 2009—Sunday

After breakfast, Joe went outside with the dogs to sweep leaves. Even though the leaves made a mess, it gave Joe something to do.

December 30, 2009—Tuesday

Today, Joe stood looking at the pile of leaves on the porch, wondering what do with them. I told him to sweep them off the porch. He did, but that was not what he wanted to do. I guess he wanted to pick them all up, which meant I would have to go get something to put them in. He wants me to be his surgical nurse.

January 1, 2010—Friday

This Christmas and New Year's was sad. I wonder how our health will be next year.

I know there are no guarantees. Each one of us should practice living in the Now.

January 3, 2010—Sunday

Ed Burleson picked us up for lunch today. Before we left, Joe quietly came over to my chair and whispered, "Are all these people going out to eat with us?" I asked him, "What people?" He looked toward the kitchen. No one was there. I shook my head, no. He looked relieved. I wonder if he saw people. Is it his imagination, or what?

Joe and I retired before 10p.m. He immediately began asking questions. It would be wonderful to have a conversation about our day, our dinner, or anything but these questions. Joe wanted to know if I had ever lived on 17th Street. I told him, "No, I am your wife." He said he knew that. I asked him what my name was. He told me to give him a hint. I asked if Deane rang a bell. Joe told me he should have known that. Then he said, "This isn't good, it isn't safe for you, it could be dangerous." Then I asked if he was frightened. He said, yes. Just think about how you would feel not knowing who is in bed with you and not knowing where you are. I assured him he had nothing to be frightened about. "I am right by your side and that will never change," I said. He told me, "You are a good person."

This journey across the rough terrain of Alzheimer's can easily break one's spirit, but I will not let my spirit be broken. If I did, I would miss the love Joe shows me off and on throughout the day. Holding back my tears, we both fell asleep. Tomorrow is another day. I pray to God day and night to provide me with the patience and stamina to take care of Joe, forever.

January 6, 2010—Wednesday

Before we got in bed tonight, Joe asked where I was going to sleep. I told him, "I am sleeping with you, like I have for fifty-eight years, in the same bed we've slept in for forty-two years." He said he had just talked to his brother, Roy, and that Roy was sleeping with him. Roy has been dead for at least 26 years.

Joe's questions continued. It was eleven o'clock and I told him to turn his questions over to God. "That is what I do when I need help," I told him. Joe said it would be nice if it worked. I asked Joe if he believed in God, and he said, "Yes." I asked him if he believed in Jesus. "Of course I do," he said. Without saying another word, Joe immediately stopped asking questions. He had been asking questions for two hours. I had my eyes closed, and the room was very quiet— almost eerie. Twenty minutes later, I began to cry. I was so relieved and shocked that Joe's questions had stopped at the moment I suggested he let God have his problem. I was worried my tears and sniffing would alert Joe, and he would begin asking more questions. I said to myself, "Loduska, do you believe?" And I answered myself, "Yes, I do." Then I began to cough. Again, I thought the coughing would alert him. I said, "Devil, quit making me cough." I asked myself again, "Do you believe?" If I truly believed, then crying or coughing wouldn't interfere with God's plan. I opened my eyes, and looked around the room. I just knew I would see a shadow or something. I closed my eyes again. Joe was quiet. I looked around the room again, and felt only stillness. At 11:45p.m., Joe got up to go to the bathroom without asking a single question. When he got back in bed, he thanked me. I told him I didn't do anything. It was God.

I have witnessed God's messages to me, and it looks as if I still doubt. I have seen double rainbows, our room number at the hotel in Austin was "316," and I know an angel came over to visit with Mindy and I at I-Hop when we were going back for my second DBS surgery. The florist, Harry Reed, received Sweet Peas the day before I ordered the spray for my mother's casket. Harry said he had not had any sweet peas in over five years, but he got three boxes of sweet peas the day before I called my order in. God sent me the idea to do a monologue to Joe every night. This nightly monologue has shortened Joe's sun downing.

Last year, when my help told me she would not work after November 1, 2009, I knew I had to search for someone else. That same day, our daughter Dena got a call from Melissa. The lady that Melissa was working for was moving to Dallas, and Melissa needed work. I hired Melissa that day. Melissa gives me some freedom to do things just for me, and she is wonderful with Joe. Melissa was sent to us in this time of conflict to ease our stress. God has sent more messages that I don't recall. I believe there is a message for each of us every day. We have to be quiet, aware, and alert to receive the message. Most of all, we have to *listen*.

January 7, 2010—Thursday

When we were ready to get in bed tonight, Joe said he would wait for me to lead the way. The way this Alzheimer's is working on him, I shudder to think what life will be like in ten years. I will not go there. Joe is Joe, and I have faith that his memory will not take a tumble.

P.S. I continually tell myself that the Axona protein drink is going to keep him constant.

January 8, 2010—Friday

Joe roamed all day. He asked lots of questions, and seemed lost. By the time we went to our bedroom to get ready to sleep, I told him, "I don't care if you brush your teeth or take your pills." To my surprise, Joe brushed his teeth and took his pills. Maybe this is the way to handle him instead of trying to fix it all. Maybe if I quit answering Joe, he'll stop asking questions.

January 11, 2010—Monday

After lunch, I tried another pep talk with Joe. I encouraged him to practice more, and find something productive to do. After the talk, he said he should see a doctor. He has no memory of ever seeing a doctor. As a matter of fact, he has no memory of taking his pills five minutes after he swallows them.

Ed picked us up for dinner. These outings are my only lifeline to sanity. Shortly after we returned home, Joe's questions began. He said a man called him about a band job in Austin. He was mad because he didn't get the man's name and because I didn't know it either. Joe roamed for the next three hours, looking above every door for our room number. He thought we were in a hotel in Austin. He walked from room to room and also outside, looking for the stairs or an elevator so he could go downstairs. He picked up the phone to call the front desk. When he picked up the phone, the operator said, "If you want to make a call, hang up and try again." Joe thought the woman at the front desk was rude and wouldn't help him. He told me if I had any part in this mêlée he would get even with me. I told him that he scared me. I am not afraid of Joe, but when he is in the zone he is not the normal Joe I know. When I began to cry, Joe was gentle and it seemed he was leaving the "A" zone. This must have been around 8p.m. When we got in bed later, the questions didn't slow down until midnight.

I don't know how I do this night after night. If we didn't have any good times, these trips with Alzheimer's would be more difficult. But I am still deeply in love with my Joe and want him by my side.

January 13, 2010—Wednesday

I called Dena today, hoping she would be able to come over to help me. Joe was in the Al zone. We were getting ready for bed, and Dena called back. Joe and I picked up the phone at the same time. I was stressed, tired, confused, and needed to know our children would come to my rescue. I told Dena I had been handling this disease solo, and I would solo it until the end of me or Joe, and I hung up. What a laugh when I read from Alzheimer's manuals that Alzheimer's is a *family* disease. Alzheimer's is the caregiver's and the patient's disease. The family usually doesn't want to have their life interrupted, or so it seems to me. I went to bed and Joe was still talking to Dena. From his end of the conversation, I was the troubled one. Once I knew Joe was asleep, I began to cry. I am drowning in this boat alone with Alzheimer's.

January 14, 2010—Thursday

Melissa didn't come to work today. I was dreading the long day with just Joe and me. I had decided that from today on if any of our kids ever call to ask how we're doing, I am going to tell them if they really want to know, then they should drop by and see for themselves. I finally put the receiver back on the hook. I need to keep the phone line open. I may not *want* to talk to our kids and give them updates about us, but I'm sure I will continue to do so. Jody called around noon, and I told Joe I couldn't come to the phone. I talked Joe into practicing his trumpet, and we were on the way to the practice room when Jody called back. I decided to talk. I got myself together so I wouldn't cry and told Jody we were fine. Of course when Joe answered the phone, Jody could tell that Joe didn't know where he was. I told Jody in my upbeat voice (I didn't feel upbeat) that I had a coke for Joe and myself, and that we were on the way to the practice room. I said, "We are good." I have to put our kids second if I am to enjoy any part of this life. I can't dwell on what I wish from them, but will dwell on the love affair I have had with Joe all of our married life. It is the same love with cracks in the road. Alzheimer's does make big cracks. I don't know why the doctors don't call Alzheimer's what it really is . . . Alzheimer's is Cancer Of The Brain.

January 15, 2010—Friday

I am not going to dwell on our kids' indifference towards my misery. I can't change their way of thinking. I am sure that each child is worried about me and wondering how long I can keep up this pace. I wonder the same thing, but I am not going to move Joe away. Joe and I deserve to spend these last year's side by side. Jody is coming for a visit. I wish all the children knew how much emotional stability their presence means to me. The four of them are the only family Joe and I have.

Jody, Mindy, Eric, Joe and I went to Applebee's for dinner. I had to remind them to include their dad in the conversation. The kids get together and enjoy visiting, and that is the way it should be. But Joe is lost, and it is impossible for him to follow their conversation. I insist that they make him the center of the conversation. Do they really forget he is sick?

January 16, 2010—Saturday

Joe got mad at me because I refused to continue answering his questions. He told me I was crazy, that he had known for years I had a mental problem, and that now he is sure I do. He wanted to call someone to come and get him. He wanted to call the police to take him home or get me out of the house. But I didn't want him to do anything that would embarrass him when he was out of the zone.

Joe looked at the phone and said there were no numbers on the phone. Is this another piece of the puzzle?

Joe called Mindy, and she and Jim came over. Mindy gave Joe a choice of staying here in his home or going home with her. He told Mindy he thought I had a mental problem. Then he said when someone thinks another person is crazy, the accuser might have a problem himself. After talking to Joe for almost two hours, Mindy finally convinced him to get ready for bed. He didn't want me to sleep with him. Ten minutes after he was in bed, he came down the hall wanting money to buy himself coffee in the morning. Back to bed he went. Ten more minutes passed, and he was coming back down the hall wanting to know when I was coming to bed. I asked him if he wanted me to sleep with him. As quick as the blink of an eye, he was out of the zone and thought my question was silly. "Yes I want you to sleep with me. Where else would you sleep?" he said.

We were in bed by 9:30p.m., and Joe was loving and affectionate.

January 17, 2010—Sunday

Ed picked us up, and we went to eat at Red Lobster. It was taking a long time for us to be seated, so I asked the hostess if we were next on the list. She told me they just needed to clean off the table. I offered to help. She said the party had paid, but was still sitting at the table. She told me to go stare at them. I did better than that. I went to their table, and asked if they enjoyed their dinner. I said to them, "I am seventy-nine years old with bad knees, my husband has Alzheimer's, the other three in our party are old, all three are diabetic, and the other man walks with a cane." I then told them that we were anxious to eat. In less than ten minutes, the three big guys walked by us. I was very nice to the men, and honest. On their way out, they stopped and shook my hand. I thanked them. Believe it or not, they were all smiling.

January 19, 2010—Tuesday

I had to fight back my rage and resentment this morning. What do I do? How do I survive?

How do I let Joe's love for me cover up my irritation? If I know Joe truly loves me, then why do I have this resentment? My resentment is not permanent. It is very fleeting.

Tonight in bed, I refused to answer any more of Joe's questions. A short time passed. I looked over at Joe lying there with his eyes open, not even watching TV, but just looking up at the ceiling. My heart melted. I told him I would answer any questions he had. How could I be so callous? From now on, I will comfort Joe by answering his questions.

Before we fell asleep, he patted me, and said, "You are mine, all mine."

January 20, 2010—Wednesday

Joe and I had dinner at Casa with Ed and Carolyne. Joe was fine until we pulled up in front of our house. He said he didn't recognize it as our home. Joe began sun downing when we got out of Ed's car. I pointed out pictures hanging on the wall of our home, but Joe didn't buy it. At 9p.m., I suggested we go to bed. Finally, when Joe walked into our bedroom and saw his green sweater hanging on the valet, he knew he was at home. To think, a green sweater would have that kind of impact on his memory.

January 21, 2010—Thursday

Joe began his sun downing around 6p.m. I asked him if he wanted me to drive him around. We visited Mindy, and ate dinner with them. Before we left to go to Mindy's, Joe kept saying he wanted to go back to his home on south 6th Street. He was no more than twelve or thirteen when he lived on 6th. It was a down time for his family. Joe's dad was ill and had to leave the lucrative Liberty Service Station that he owned with a brother. Dissolving the partnership didn't leave the Johnson's with much. Why Joe wants to go back to 1941, I don't know. Was that a time when he was secure?

January 22, 2010—Friday

This morning, I asked Joe if he had the newspaper, and he said he did. I picked up the paper he was reading, and realized it was yesterday's paper. He didn't know the difference. As I was going to the front porch to get today's paper, I said to myself, "God, get this chip off my shoulder and let only kind, loving words come from my lips."

Joe spent the afternoon raking leaves.

We had not finished dinner before Joe began saying he wanted to go home. I told him we were at home. This went on for an hour or more. Joe gets frustrated when I don't give him the answers he wants. Then I am the one who is crazy, and he starts saying he doesn't know why he ever got mixed up with me. The look in his eyes is scary. I can't help crying. I want to help him. I want to scream at him! I want to tell him to go to hell, but using those words with a sharp tone of voice would put him deeper into his "A" zone. I don't want to ever use a harsh tone. I love him too much to act unloving.

This evening, I talked Joe into practicing his horn, but it didn't last. He thought I told him to get his horn because he was going to play a job. I called Dena, and asked her to tell Joe where he was. They talked a minute or two, and Joe hung up. I knew that meant I was on my own with this Joe I slightly fear.

About that time, I heard Dena's voice, the voice of an Angel, and she came in and sat by Joe. She brought pictures of her family. Joe appeared to be interested, but continued telling us he wanted to go home.

Dena suggested we take a ride, and Joe asked if she would take him home. She said, "Let's go get in my car." Joe took his trumpet, and we all piled in the car.

Dena took us all around Waco. On the way home, she pointed out that this was the way he always came home from the court house for forty years. He agreed. Dena stopped at the street signs so he could read the street sign. She got us in the house, and Joe was ready to turn in. He was still a bit skeptical about our whereabouts, but sleep finally moved in. I just wonder how many more of these kinds of nights I can handle if I have to do it alone.

January 23, 2010—Saturday

The day was smooth until the ol' Al zone visited Joe. I buckled down for more of the same questions. In these moments, Joe never hesitates to tell me I'm crazy. I called Mindy, and Jim answered. I asked him if he would drop by for thirty minutes. He and Mindy were both here in less than thirty minutes. I had managed to get Joe calmed down some before they arrived. Mindy and Jim were on the way to the twins' (Jackson & Eric) senior prom to take pictures. After the conversation about the boys, Joe was almost in the "now" by the time they left.

January 24, 2010—Sunday

I finally got Joe to practice his trumpet. I bet he oiled the valves at least five times. I think that was his way of postponing the practice. He practiced for about an hour. I called out tunes, and, without any hesitation, he played the song. Joe makes that trumpet sing. Alzheimer's may block some of his memory, but not his musical memory.

January 25, 2010—Monday

After a short time of me being on the computer, Joe came in the room in his underwear looking for me.

His demeanor was the same as a two or three-year old looking for their mother. Truthfully, I have to admit it doesn't make me feel special. I know I am responsible for helping him get dressed, brush his teeth, and making his breakfast while keeping a smile on my face. This is another day of care giving.

I made Joe and myself a sandwich for lunch. He looked just like a child, with a smile on his face, sitting in his place at the bar waiting for his lunch.

Joe did not sun down at all today, but he was slightly lost when we went to bed. He wasn't sure where the bedroom was. If only every day was like today—fairly calm and no sun downing.

January 27, 2010—Wednesday

After dinner, I began talking to Joe about something that happened today. I still forget he doesn't remember enough things that happen throughout the day to be capable of having any kind of conversation. For me to come face to face with this reality every day is a downer. I hate to admit that I am not nice. How can he forget what happened an hour ago? Joe began reminiscing in bed tonight. I don't know if he was reminiscing or talking about how he felt at that moment. He talked about what a good sex life we've had, how close we have been since the beginning of our marriage, and he complemented our long relationship as loving with few disagreements. I don't care if he remembers these fifty-eight years or if he is talking about today. His conversation was calming and rewarding. When this happens, I don't question him. I just marvel in the moment.

January 27, 2010—Wednesday

Dear Dr. Morledge,

Some days I think I see a difference in Joe. Today about all I can say is that Joe is mellower than usual. When he sun downs (which is most every day), he isn't in the zone as long. Most days I can sweet talk him out of the zone back into the present moment. Then there are days I have to call one of our daughters over to the house to help bring him back to his right mind.

It is getting harder to get him to practice the trumpet. Today I talked to him directly about the decline he will reach much faster if he doesn't use his brain. We went to the practice room, and Joe played for an hour. When he puts the trumpet to his lips, he enjoys playing. I called out tunes, and he played each and every one without any hesitation.

All that said, thank you for your encouragement, your understanding, and for being in the wings for Joe and me.

Lovingly,
Deane Johnson

January 29, 2010—Friday

I left the house for a little while this afternoon, and when I got back home, Joe didn't even know I had left. After he ate lunch, he began to roam. He started out the front door with the trash, but the trash isn't picked up until Monday. Joe wanted to check the faucets outside in case of a freeze. He would not sit down all day.

January 31, 2010—Sunday

Joe had a little sun downing when going to bed tonight. I kept repeating, "We are at home, and I am your wife." When I get tired of repeating myself, I show him the card where I wrote, "We are at home." He reads it as if this is the first time he has seen it. At times, I just refuse to believe that he cannot remember. *Alzheimer's* is a very dirty word, a death sentence taking Joe further and further away from me. If I am not careful, I will fall in this hole and cry until the end. I remember when we used to stay up late and talk, and perhaps have some intimate time before sleep moved in. That was yesterday. This is today.

I must learn to enjoy the moment, and tuck all of our yesterday's away safely in my memory diary. My memories will be a trip to our past with Joe by my side. I will make good memories every day. Chin up ol' gal, there are good days ahead.

February 4, 2010—Thursday

Every time Joe comes in the kitchen and sits at the bar wanting to be waited on, I want to scream at him. I don't want to be a maid. I don't want to be responsible for getting out his clothes, fixing his meals, ordering and dispensing his pills, taking us to exercise, getting him to shower, shave, and brush his teeth, taking care of all the investments, paying the bills, keeping cars gassed and running, and being his recreation director. I know Joe appreciates all I do. I know without me he wouldn't have a clue about anything. I know this is my job. I wish I didn't resent doing these things. I do find pleasure being Joe's wife. But the roles have changed. I have to change too, and I am trying. At times, I want out. But that feeling is fleeting. If I wasn't here with Joe, I would be miserable. My advice to me is in the title of the song, "*Straighten Up And Fly Right.*"

Joe began sun downing just before we went to bed. He wanted to know his mother's phone number and where the cars were. Sleep overtook him by 11p.m.

February 5, 2010—Friday

Joe feels alone and lonely throughout the day and evening. When he asked about his mom last night, he didn't remember her funeral. He questioned me, wondering why I hadn't told him about it. That is lonely.

At the grocery store, Joe is always polite, speaks to most people, and tells the ladies they are pretty. He doesn't want to get in front of anyone's basket.

When we got in bed tonight, Joe began to sing "I Love You Truly" and "I Left my Heart in San Francisco." I had never heard him sing these songs before, but he certainly knew the tune and remembered most of the words. The mind is a remarkable tool, even with Alzheimer's.

P.S. My granddaughter, Stacy, is twenty today. Our grandbabies are growing up.

February 8, 2010—Monday

I was watching TV this afternoon when Joe quickly got up to go to the bathroom. When he returned, I asked him if he had made it to the potty in time, and he shook his head.

I am so tired of the unrelenting responsibilities I have every day. When I complain, Joe doesn't think I have much to do. The only thing he knows is what is happening at the moment. He doesn't remember even when I tell him. When I am being "poor Deane," I tell him how much I do for him. It doesn't do any good, but it at least allows me to vent.

February 10, 2010—Wednesday

Joe and I were sitting in the den around 6p.m., I was reading a book and our conversation went something like this:

Joe: Honey, I love you. You are mine, all mine. Do you love me?
Deane: (I nod and continue reading)
Joe: I guess she doesn't love me!
Deane: Joe, I nodded, yes. I take care of your needs all day every day. The things I do for you should show you the deep love I have for you. I took you to see Dr. Stern this morning to get a shot for your back and—
Joe (interrupting): Did I go to the doctor this morning? I don't remember it, if I did.

He then waited to follow me back to our bedroom again. Nothing looks familiar to him. When we got in bed, he began to talk about his mother again, saying how much he missed her. I wish I could say or do the right thing to comfort him.

I hate to admit that this disease is not only whipping Joe, but I am getting a whipping too. My husband is slowly slipping away. One thing I must do is make an effort to appreciate all his questions. The day may come quicker than I expect when he won't ask me questions anymore. Boy, would I hate for this disease to go there. I will enjoy this time with Joe, because who knows what tomorrow may bring.

February 11, 2010—Thursday

My tears stay under control unless I hear a comforting voice. My tears are always just under the surface, and if I perceive a kind, caring, loving tone in a friend's or family member's voice or eyes, I cry. What I really want to do is put my head down and not just cry, but scream. I am afraid that if I start, I may never stop.

P.S. Today, Joe practiced his trumpet while I wrote in my journal.

February 12, 2010—Friday

There is a little snow on the ground, and it is very cold today. I began trying to get Joe up around 11p.m. He wouldn't budge. It dawned on me that Joe might not get up because he doesn't know where he is. I kept urging him to get up, and he called to me for help because his back hurt. He had no memory that his back hurt yesterday too, or that he had received a shot on Wednesday. As far as he remembered, his back had just begun to hurt this morning.

This afternoon, Joe was acting like he was in the early years of Alzheimer's. We were having a conversation, and he was worried about me. He told me if he ever began to fall just to let him fall so I wouldn't get hurt. Logic! For a moment, I wondered if Joe was recovering some of his memory.

Later, Joe came in the room wanting to know where the hearing was, thinking he was still an active Judge. He looked out the window to see if he could see anyone. How dumb of me to think Joe might recover some of his memory. I royally set myself up for disappointment with that thought.

This has been a long, dreary day. I wrote some on the computer, and Joe came in the office to see what I was doing. He left acting forlorn, because I didn't jump up and go back to the den with him. His back hurt and he wanted instant relief, so I finally went in the den to sit with him.

February 13, 2010—Saturday

There is a song title, *"How Long Has This Been Going On?"* It seems longer than six years since Joe was diagnosed. No one has any idea what it is like living with Alzheimer's.

February 14, 2010—Sunday

Email to family:

Dear Family,
    I took the trash out and when I came back in the house Joe was lying on the floor. He had attempted to climb over the doggy gate, and had fallen. He assured me he was okay. About an hour later, I heard him calling for me. He had gone to the half bath, which has a step up. His leg had given out, and he was lodged in the door. I finally got him up off the ground so he could pee. What a day!

Love,
Deane

Reply from our niece, Stacey:

    So sorry about Uncle Joe's fall! It worries me that this may start being more frequent. My heart is with all of you. Love, Stacey

February 22, 2010—Monday

We have reached the point that I can't be alone with Joe in his physical and mental condition. I will stay strong in order to keep Joe with me.

February 23, 2010—Tuesday

    Joe was up at 6a.m., delusional. I tried to get him to rest, but he was mentally out of it. I finally got up to take a shower. The look in Joe's eyes was a warning to me not to get myself cornered in the bathroom. He was still in the bed, so I locked the door to take a shower. Soon, Joe began knocking on the door. I told him I was showering. In his delusion, and this was very real to him, he saw me having sex with a man in our bathroom. At this point, I was afraid of Joe. I called Mindy, and she came right over. Melisa Mercer from Visiting Angels wasn't due until 11a.m. Mindy tried to reason with

Joe. I didn't attempt to talk to him because he was angry with me, still thinking I had been unfaithful. He stared at me and moved his hand across his throat, as if to say I was a dead woman. He was certain that what he had seen was real, even though it was an illusion in his mind. Joe zoned the rest of the day.

Mindy picked me up, and we went over to see the Alzheimer's Care home on N. 19th. Sabreena, the Resident Nurse (RN), mentioned that a bladder infection could be the cause of Joe having delusions. The facility was like a residence. There was a large den, a dining room, an open kitchen, a large covered porch, and a fenced yard. The individual rooms opened to a hall circling the main room. At this time, there are six patients. I was shown a room, and it was nice. I sat down on the bed, covered my face, and cried like a big baby. I can't face the thought of moving Joe to live apart from me.

February 25, 2010—Thursday

I took Joe to get a pedicure today. He always enjoys seeing John, the manager, and getting a pedicure. I sat and watched Joe enjoying his pedicure, and wondered how many more times this would happen. I don't think I am courageous enough to place Joe in the Alzheimer's Care home right now. What would that do to him, and what would it do to me? Would I cry just looking at his empty chair and his empty spot in the bed? How would I deal with his absence all around the house? How do I even begin to go there?

February 26, 2010—Friday

At breakfast with Joe, I brought up the idea of assisted living. When we began talking about him moving, he was agreeable, but then he was unsure. Joe is as unsure of a move as I am. When we got in bed, he began questioning me about things that need to get done. It was as if he wanted to be sure I knew what to do if he wasn't here with me. He wanted to be sure I kept my license up to date on the car. Then he asked where I would get money if I needed it. Lastly, he asked who I would call to ask for money if I was out of town. He then told me he hoped our kids would look after me. It is as if he knows I am going to move him away from me. I will not move Joe. If I did, I would need medication to survive the days alone.

February 27, 2010—Saturday

Earlier today, Joe was outside picking up twigs, and he fell. He said he thought he had experienced a stroke. I called Mindy. Laura (who was here when Joe fell) called her husband to pick up Joe. We did not take Joe to the hospital, even though he wanted to go. Mindy and I were satisfied that Joe had not blacked out, and decided his leg had just given way and had caused him to fall.

At dinner, Joe and I discussed him making another CD. He was logical to the point of telling me that he will make the CD for me. I hope he will. I don't want to put Joe in a home. At this point in time, I won't do it.

March 2, 2010—Tuesday

When I got home from running errands this afternoon, Joe was mad. He told Melisa Mercer that he thought I was meeting with another man. Joe said if he had a gun, he would shoot the other guy. Joe was uneasy for some time. When he is in the zone, I am ready to move him, but that feeling doesn't last long enough for me to follow through.

March 6, 2010—Saturday

Joe and I had a long talk about the assisted living home. He stayed on the subject for about three hours. At one point, we were sitting in our chairs, and Joe looked at me and asked, "*Are you going to move me away from the only woman I've ever loved?*" That question broke my heart. At this time, I am not strong enough to make any kind of decisions about Joe or myself.

March 7, 2010—Sunday

As we sat watching the Academy Awards tonight, Joe told me over and over to be quiet because I was interfering with the host on TV. Joe can't separate reality from the TV. He thought the show was happening in our den.

March 8, 2010—Monday

Tommy Ledbetter, Joe's cousin called me today, and encouraged me to place Joe in the assisted living. I told him what Joe said about moving him from the only woman he had ever loved. Tommy's reply was, "Oh yes, even in their mental state the person with AD can still make one feel guilty." He warned me that Joe may get physically violent as the disease progresses. He said his law partner, Max, was in his seventh year before he began to grab his wife.

I know, I know, I thought.

But I can't take Joe away to assisted living at this stage. He is still the loving Joe I've always known, but simply without any purpose in his life. He still appreciates whatever is done for him, even though he offers to do nothing for others. He has no incentive. It is as if he knows he should be doing something but doesn't know what he should do. That is why he often asks if I need help. I usually just thank him, and tell him I'm fine.

March 14, 2010—Sunday

Ed called this afternoon, and we met the group at Olive Garden. Joe began to sun down right after we returned home. This went on until at least 2a.m. Joe thought he was at Baylor University for a little while, and wild animals were roaming around. Then he thought he was at a carnival. When Joe is in the zone, he communicates clearly what he sees in his mind. At one point, Joe woke me up, hovering over me, so that a so-called statue wouldn't fall on me. I felt his arms over my head, and it startled me.

March 19, 2010—Friday

When I was on the computer this evening, Joe came in the room ordering me to turn it off. I did as he requested, just to appease him. Did I like it? Hell no, I didn't like it. Later, I was watching TV in the bed, and he wanted the TV off. I guess I am a prisoner in my own home, but I'll do almost anything to cut down the sun-downing. I was irritated. Joe talked until midnight.

March 20, 2010—Saturday

Joe didn't get up until almost noon today. This is what his first half hour of the day looked like:

1. I got him to brush his teeth. (He just stood with a blank look on his face)
2. I put out his clothes. (He put them on)
3. I reminded him to get his glasses. (He didn't know where they were)
4. I fixed his Axona drink, breakfast, and coffee. (He sat waiting to be pampered)
5. I had to sit with him, and I didn't want to.

This is as good as Joe is going to be. I find myself wanting to distance myself from him, though I am not yet ready to take him to the Alz home. I ask myself, *What do you want, Deane?* The fact of the matter is that I love Joe, and I don't want to push him away. I know he needs me now more than ever, and I need him too, just in a different way. I need my space just as much as he does. I have to get in my cocoon in order to survive. Once I take some time for me, it is easier to be Joe's caregiver. When I leave his side, he feels alone. Joe would like for me to sit at the bar or in a chair across from him all day until bedtime. I know I can't do that while maintaining a pleasant aura. I am well aware that being an only child is the reason for my need to have private time. Joe came from a large family. Being the baby of the family, he was always surrounded with siblings and parents who pampered him in his early years. I didn't have that, so I pampered myself in my own fantasy world.

March 21, 2010—Sunday

Sometimes Joe will whistle in his sleep. Last night, he whistled a tune from beginning to end while he slept. I wish I could remember the tune. When he is dreaming in the zone, he talks very distinctly. Last night in his dreams, he was busy with the Texas Rangers.

When I am soloing, I have to fight my resentment toward Joe. I wish I could be a better person. I wish it was easier to be kind and loving while I am getting him up, putting out his clothes, making his breakfast, and answering all his questions at least twice. An outsider would probably think I don't love him, but that's not true. I love the Joe of yesterday, and I love the Alzheimer's Joe, but his condition weighs heavily on both him and me.

March 22, 2010—Monday

Tonight, Joe woke up and thought he was the Fire Marshall. I guess he thought he saw people sitting in chairs in the den, because he questioned the imaginary men until 6a.m. Joe's questions were, "Who set the fire?" "Can't any of you talk?" "I'm not going to hurt you. I am Joe Johnson, answer me." His diction was perfect, and his vocabulary was very good. I hid the car keys in case he tried to leave the house.

March 23, 2010—Tuesday

I had to get out of the house today. I went to get my allergy shot, and when I walked in, my tears were uncontrollable. The girls put me in a private room, and several girls and Dr. Daftary spent time with me. When I am this tired, I am ready to move Joe to the Alz Care home. But before I take my next breath, I can't bring myself to put him in a home.

I lay in the bed tonight praying and trying to figure out what would be the best for Joe and for me. Why does it take me so long to get God's message? I am not in control. I can't fix my life and Joe's life. I turned this worry and decision over to God. Gosh, it was a weight off my shoulders. I can't believe I chose to carry this burden while God was waiting to take my burdens all along. I fell asleep, and slept through the entire night without any interruptions.

March 24, 2010—Wednesday

When I woke up this morning, I felt like a free person—no guilt, no worry, just peace. I gave these worries and decisions to God.

March 27, 2010—Saturday

Joe began singing hymns tonight. He didn't know all the words. We sang *The Old Rugged Cross* and *Amazing Grace*. He whistled *How Great Thou Art*. Every night, Joe and I say the Lord's Prayer and the Apostles' Creed aloud.

After we sang for a while, Joe asked me where his horse was. I told him he's never had a horse. He said that he had had a horse. I don't know what part of his past that statement came from, but I had to laugh. We slept all night.

March 28, 2010—Sunday

I wonder if we will ever go to church again. I don't think Joe would last through the service. This is another solo day for me.

Tonight around 8p.m., Joe didn't know where he was, where the cars were, or how we got here in this house. He began asking me when we were going to go home and who owned this "building." It is hard to comprehend that while we were eating, Joe knew where we were. And then a couple hours later, he was lost again. Eventually, he got out of bed and sat in the easy chair, still not knowing where he was.

Every night is a bad dream for me. My husband of 58 years is missing. I can't reach him when he is in the zone, and I am so alone even when Joe is in the same room sitting across from me. At times, this is a nightmare.

March 31, 2010—Wednesday

Melissa was late this morning. She didn't get here until almost noon. After I woke up, I showered, and then went to the kitchen for my coffee and to read the newspaper. I finally got Joe up and fixed his Axona drink, a sandwich, orange juice, and coffee.

April 4, 2010—Easter Sunday

At times, I feel sorry for myself. I don't ask much from Joe at all. Today, I told Joe I don't ask much of him. He listened, and said he was sorry to cause me to feel that way. He got up and showered, shampooed, and even shaved and brushed his teeth. Luckily, when I am honest with Joe, he leaves the zone.

April 5, 2010—Monday

This morning, I asked Joe how he was feeling, and he asked me if I had worked lately. He called me Billy.
I said, "Billy who?"
He answered, "Billy Johnson." A trumpet player from his past.
"Do I look like Billy Johnson?" I asked.
He said yes, and then he called me Iva.
Joe didn't know who I was until the middle of the afternoon.

April 7, 2010—Wednesday

I talked Joe into practicing his trumpet today. Once he got started, he enjoyed the session. I called out a song from the list for his next

CD, and he played the song from beginning to end in his own style. Joe is amazing, a talent from God, and his own creative improvisation is a wonder to my ears. I pray he will always be able to play the trumpet and sing.

When I suggested we go to bed, Joe again had no idea where our bedroom was.

April 10, 2010—Saturday

Dena visited today, and Joe and I both enjoyed her being here with us. Joe played his trumpet for a little while. Then he sang "It Had to be You," making up lyrics when he forgot what came next. I wish I had recorded his rendition of the song. The lyrics he made up were not just good, they were meaningful.

April 11, 2010—Sunday

When I get up in the mornings, I talk to myself about keeping my resentment under control.

Every day seems the same as the day before. But I can either look at today as more of the same, or I can choose to relish each moment I have with Joe.

Barry stopped by to visit this afternoon. He finds humor in all his surroundings. When he visits, it is like having a front row seat to the show of an outstanding comedian. If he is depressed, and he has every reason to be, no one would ever know it. His humor is a gift to us, and his visits just don't happen often enough.

April 12, 2010—Monday

I went to the dentist after Melissa got here at 11a.m. I had lost a crown, and felt I deserved to have a new one that will last me until the time comes for me to move to my next home in Oakwood Cemetery. Surprisingly, Joe remembered how I feel about visits to the dentist. It is amazing that he may forget who I am at times, but he remembers how I have always feared the dentist. Figure that.

April 15, 2010—Thursday

Our grandsons, Jackson and Eric, dropped by for a visit and to pick up some jackets for a party they were going to. We enjoyed their visit. Joe knew who they were. He conversed with the boys, and I could tell he didn't want me entering into the conversation while he had the floor. I gave them two shirts that we wore when Joe was running for the 170th District Judge. Joe has been known to be selfish with his clothes, but he was happy that the boys wanted to wear his shirts.

Joe had no idea where our bedroom was when we were ready to retire for the night. When we got in the bedroom, he did recognize our bed.

April 17, 2010—Saturday

This afternoon, Joe shaved and got dressed for his band job tonight. I told Ed to go ahead and hire Byron in case Joe got tired of playing. I gave Ed money to pay Joe. I didn't think it was fair for Ed to pay two trumpet players, and I wanted Joe to get his pay envelope at the end of the job. This job is as much for me as it is for Joe. This may be his last job. With this disease, one never knows. I will encourage him to play as long as he is able to play, and as long as he wants to. When Joe puts that trumpet to bed, it will be bittersweet remembering that it was his music that I fell in love with before setting eyes on him, but it will not end my love affair with Joe. Joe's music will fill my mind and heart forever.

In 1950, before I ever walked in the ballroom and saw Joe on the bandstand at Casa Blanca, I heard the trumpet solo, and then heard the vocalist singing. I walked to the door and saw Joe at the microphone singing with his trumpet in hand. I fell in love with Joe that night. Now, 59 years later, I am still in love with the man with the horn.

Mindy picked us up at 5p.m. today to go to the Shrine band job. Joe played a four-hour job and never once complained about his lip. He played every tune and also sang the blues. It was amazing watching him laugh and cut up with Byron and Aubrey who play in the band. It has been a long time since Joe had any guy time. Joe's contact with the outside world is limited these days.

On the way home, he didn't know where we were going. Also, he knew he had been paid, but he forgot he put the envelope in his shirt pocket. Joe was confused when we got home. He wanted to go to his own home. He was tired when we finally went to bed. He went right to sleep, but soon woke up. There is one thing still in his memory, and it is sex after playing a job. Joe was not able to consummate the sex act this time. Consummate or not, to cuddle and be intimate with Joe was enough for us both.

April 18, 2010—Sunday

We watched golf most of the day. Later in the afternoon, Joe picked up the broom and began sweeping. When it came time to put out the trash, Joe was frustrated. There was too much for him to put in order: opening the gates, pulling two trash cans to the curb, and closing the gates. Overall, the day almost felt like things were back to normal. We retired around 10p.m.

April 21, 2010—Wednesday

Joe was totally lost when he woke up this morning. He didn't know me, and he wanted me to leave. I sat outside with Joe, hoping to calm him and reassure him. I eventually came in the house. In less than five minutes, Joe came too. The zone stayed outside. When Joe walked in the back door, he knew who I was, and he was loving and calm. Yes, going in and out of the zone is as quick as the bat of an eye.

April 29, 2010—Thursday

This morning, Joe was anxious because he couldn't find me. If I am in another room and he doesn't hear me, he thinks he is alone.

Joe and I went out for pancakes. A lady stopped by our table to say hello. I suspected her husband might have Alzheimer's. She knew Joe from the court house. As she was leaving the restaurant, she said to me, "God bless you." I knew then her husband had Alzheimer's, and she knew Joe had Alzheimer's. Looking at her husband in the mental stage he was in, I knew right then I would never take Joe out in public if he wasn't dressed nicely and clean. If Joe has that faraway look in his eye and he is in the kind of mental state her husband was in, I don't think we would go out at all. When we returned home, the questions began. At times, Joe is impossible, or maybe it is that I am at the end of my rope. I feel like I am sinking in quicksand—not with Alzheimer's, but with the burden of Alzheimer's. Tonight, I thought that I was ready to send Joe to Alz Care. I tried to get Joe to shower, but in his frame of mind he wasn't going to do anything that I wanted him to do. I thought, "To hell with it," and we both got in bed. As soon as Joe got in bed, he began telling me that I am his, all his. The zone was gone. Joe was pleased that he didn't get in the shower.

April 30, 2010—Friday

After breakfast, Joe went outside with the dogs, and I went to the computer. About an hour later, I went out to get Joe to come in so we could have a sandwich together. He was mad, because he thought I had left the house. He said he came in looking for me, and I wasn't anywhere to be found. I knew it wasn't true. He told me always to write him a note to tell him what room I'm in. But if he can't even find our bed at night, he surely couldn't find me in the office on the computer. He wouldn't know what room was our office.

May 1, 2010—Saturday

I know we won't even try to go to church tomorrow. My legs and knees hurt badly, and Joe is slow and doesn't get around too good. It would take us a long time just to get out of the car and across the street.

May 4, 2010—Tuesday

Today, Dr. Morledge emphasized daily exercise for Joe. We must stretch at least five times a week, ride the bicycle for fifteen minutes, and maybe when Melissa is here, she and Joe can take a short walk. We are going back to Super Slow too. Mindy filmed our visit with Dr. Morledge, and she will film Joe when he begins recording his next CD.

Mindy and Joe talked nearly all the way back from Austin to Waco. I know Mindy was tired, but Joe enjoyed every word they exchanged. I don't think I talk to Joe as much as I should. I know he needs a lot more conversation than I give him.

At 5p.m., Joe wanted us to go to the Piccadilly. We haven't had a Piccadilly in Waco for over ten years. It is strange that Joe thinks he has to eat, even when he is not hungry.

May, 5, 2010—Wednesday

A few nights ago, Joe and I went out to dinner. I had given him his wallet before we left home. I knew he had money in it, because I had found the cash in an envelope and had put it back in his wallet. Joe opened his wallet to pay, and it was empty. I felt sorry for him, because he looked embarrassed and belittled. I guess he had hid his money.

May 7, 2010—Friday

An old friend called today, and I could tell he had been drinking. I don't understand alcoholics. Joe talked to him, but it was not Alzheimer's Joe. Joe sounded as if he was sitting in his office at the court house. When he hung up, he asked me why I was drunk. He never did understand that it was not me. Joe told me what a no-good person I was and how sorry I was to get drunk. All evening long, he asked me to go home. We finally went to bed around 9p.m.

Joe used a forceful, controlling voice to make me turn off the television and my bed lamp. He thought we were sleeping in the First Presbyterian Church and that the police would be coming by during the night to check the premises. Joe was warning me that we would be put in jail if the police found us hiding in the church. He wanted me out of the bed, and out of the house.

I thought to myself, *You have no idea how bad I would love to get out of this house.*

I got up and went to another bedroom. I lay in bed awake, listening for him to come down the hall looking for me. Once I was sure he was asleep, I got back in my bed with Joe. If the normal Joe had woken up while I was in the other room, he would have started looking for me.

I want Joe to stay asleep. I need my sleep to face whatever my day is like tomorrow.

May 8, 2010—Saturday

Joe began insulting me this evening. I called Mindy, and she said she would come over. Instead of sitting in my chair being insulted, I got up and sat on the front porch to wait for Mindy. That was the worst thing I could have done. When I came back in, Joe was in the hall coming from our bedroom. Because he couldn't find me, he began accusing me of looking for men. Joe even insulted Mindy.

Mindy finally got him to go to bed. I had to stay out of Joe's sight, because whenever he saw me, he would call me a whore and give me the finger. Joe finally got in bed, but he told me he thought he was in jail.

After hearing his statement, I thought, *that is exactly where he is—in jail, with the albatross of Alzheimer's chocking the life out of him and Mindy and me.*

Later, Joe wanted to go to the bathroom, but he said he was afraid to get up because the sheriff might shoot him. Joe hollered "Sheriff!" several times to alert the sheriff not to shoot because he was just going to the bathroom. Mindy spent the night with us.

May 9, 2010—Sunday

Happy Mother's Day to me, Dena, and Mindy. How do we get up with a smile on our faces after all the accusations and insults we got from Joe last night? Instead, we smile with a heavy heart because we know Joe would never say those things if he was Joe without Alzheimer's.

May 10, 2010—Monday

Today, I told Joe about him being verbally abusive to me on Saturday night. He told me he would never do anything to hurt me. When his thoughts are blocked and he goes in the zone, he has no control over what he says or does. I confess I am hurt by his accusations, even though I know I shouldn't be. Joe said, "Honey, I would never hurt you. I guess you need to have feelings of steel." I wish I could. I am too sensitive, too much of a cry baby, and I love Joe too much. This is taking more of a toll on me than it is on Joe.

I went to Colby's Birthday party, and Joe was suspicious of me leaving the house. I called him a couple of times, and every time he asked me if I was with other men.

May 11, 2010—Tuesday

Joe and I were watching Glenn Beck, and Joe said I was having an affair with Beck. I kept explaining that Beck was in New York, and that we were watching him on TV. But when the zone takes over Joe's brain, nothing can change his mind. No one can get through to him.

Joe got up, pointed his finger at me and began telling me what a no good wife I was. We went out in the back yard, and I hoped a change of scenery would snap him back to reality. Joe began pacing in the yard, trying to find a way out. I called Mindy, and asked her if she had the papers filled out for the Alz Care Home. I told her what was going on. She came right over.

Seeing Mindy didn't change Joe's mind. He walked around the

fence line looking for a gate to get out and walk home. Mindy and I didn't know what to do, or how we could stop him. Joe said if he couldn't find a gate, he would jump the fence. Finally, I called Jody, Dena, and Barry to tell them we were going to begin making arrangements to move Joe.

May 12, 2010—Wednesday

I did make the decision to move Joe, but it really was a message from God. I am not, nor have ever been, strong. Since I made the decision to move Joe, I haven't been able to stop crying. I cried in the doctor's office today, and I called Ed to tell him to find a different trumpet player for Thursday night. Joe might be able to play, but it would be too emotional for me listening to Joe play for what might be his last time.

Mindy began reading and filling out the papers for the Alz Care home.

I got in bed beside Joe, knowing that I have only one more night after tonight. Sadness doesn't even begin to describe how I feel. This is the end of us being together and sleeping together, and it is a nightmare of the worse kind. It is an empty, sickening sadness that engulfs me. This is the end of our marriage as we know it.

May 13, 2010—Thursday

I sat at the bar with Joe at breakfast, but I had to look away from him. I cannot control my tears. Joe doesn't even notice I am crying. If he notices anything, he thinks I have bad allergies or a cold. I wonder how I can send my Joe away to live apart from me and also keep my sanity. But how do I continue taking care of Joe and not lose my sanity and my health? When Joe was trying to find a way out of the back yard, I knew that if he wondered off and we couldn't find him that would be worse than him living apart from me.

Mindy picked me up for lunch, and I bought pastries for Joe's breakfast tomorrow morning. It will be his last meal at home with me.

Am I strong enough to see this through? Mindy and I finished filling out the necessary papers to move Joe to his new home. That sounds awful. This will always be his home. His home is here with me, even if he sleeps somewhere else.

I wanted Melissa to cook a roast for Joe. Roast is a favorite of his. She cooked the roast in pieces. Joe asked, "What kind of roast is this?"

I think Joe may have sensed something when he got in bed tonight. He kissed me again and again. "Just one more kiss," he kept saying. Joe told me over and over how much he loved me, and then he said we shared the same heart. I told him we definitely shared the same heart. I asked if he knew who I was. Joe said, "No, but I feel very close to you." I had prayed to God to help keep my tears under control. I didn't cry. I just held Joe, thanking God for the life we've shared. I will cry the rest of my life, alone.

An e mail I sent to family and close friends on May 13, 2010:

Dear Family and Friends,

The day I have been avoiding for more than a year has come.

Mindy and I have made the necessary, heart-wrenching decision to move Joe to an Alz Care Home.

I know if I continue trying to care for Joe at home, I am destined to hit a concrete wall, and my health and sanity will be compromised if it isn't already.

I am sick with grief. This long goodbye over the past seven years has been so much stress on me and our children. I think a trip to Oakwood Cemetery wouldn't be any more stressful. I can't stop crying. I have to hide my tears from Joe, but when he sees me crying, it doesn't register. Joe thinks I have a cold. Mindy, Dena and Melissa are taking Joe to Alz Care tomorrow afternoon. I just can't go. I have to put my hands over my face to keep from screaming.

This is the most heart wrenching journey anyone could be on. I love, I cry, and I pray-pray-pray for strength to find the courage to do what needs to be done, enjoy the good times as they come, and if I can stay positive and love with all my heart maybe my heart won't break.

Love to each of you. Love your mates. Have multiple conversations, sit quietly and hold hands. Savor each other.

Deane Johnson

May 14, 2010—Friday

This is the day Joe moves. I have tried to avoid this day for over a year. I can't keep from crying. I wonder how I am going to be able to see it through.

Carolyne and Verda picked me up around 2p.m. Mindy was helping me to the car, and I almost crumbled. I couldn't breathe. I couldn't see. All I could do was fight a wave of sadness flooding over me like a tsunami.

Mindy, Dena, and Melissa took Joe to his new home. The girls had the room decorated, and his new chair had been delivered. Joe looked around the room and said it was plain. The girls left before Melissa. When Mindy and Dena got to their car, they fell apart. I am not as brave as my girls are.

Jackson and Eric came over to be with me. Stacy came by too. Mindy came by, and we all piled up in chairs for some quiet healing time. I went out to eat dinner with my daughter, the grandkids, and Jim. Mindy spent the night with me. Joe called Mindy. He was upset—probably sun downing. This is not going to be easy.

Even though my heart will be broken, Alz Care is second best to being home with me. Joe will adjust before I do. Joe likes to be around people, and the girls who work at Alz Care will take good care of him. I am thankful there is an Alz Care.

May 14, 2010—Friday

E mail to friends:

Dear Friends,

This isn't easy. I cannot stop crying. I know I can no longer keep on this pace I've been on for over seven years. I can't look any further down the road than today. When thinking about this journey, adjusting, trying to live joyfully, loving Joe every minute, reinforcing our love to him when I visit, and being without him is more than I can take in. I have been losing Joe, saying goodbye in tiny baby steps, for eight years. At first, I didn't realize we were saying goodbye. It was gradual, but now the boulder has pushed me down and under. I have to crawl out, but how?

Every night around 8p.m., Joe starts sun downing. He wants to call home. Mindy and Dena get the calls. I just can't do that every night. Facing tragedies at the end of life is something no one prepares themselves for.

Love And Prayers,
Deane Johnson

Dicque's response to my e mail:

Deane,

I guess the day has come. I feel such sympathy for you after learning about your decision that I am almost physically in pain thinking of what you are going through.

I'm so sorry, dear one. This is worse than Oakwood, but if it doesn't work for you and for Joe, you can always bring him back home.

Love You and Worry About You,
Dicque

E mail from Tommy:

God Bless you! And God Bless Joe! What else can I say? I know you shed many of your famous great big tears before you made the decision. Remember this: there is no one who loves Joe more than you, there is nothing you would not do for him, and there is nothing that anyone could do better or more caringly for him than you. What you have done for him is therefore the best that anyone could do—and it will always be enough, even though you may sometimes doubt it.

Love Ya,
Tommy

May 15, 2010—Saturday

I don't think the reality of this trauma has hit me yet.

May 16, 2010—Sunday

This day began with tears and no sunshine. There isn't anything for me to be happy about. I spent the day crying. Emotionally, I don't know how I am going to be able to visit Joe. I want to hug him and tell him everything is going to be fine. First, I have to convince myself that this separation is going to be fine. I watched TV, I wrote in my journal, and I was sadder than I thought was possible.

Ed, Carolyne, and Verda picked me up, and we had dinner. I know I'm not good company. Mindy spent the night. Joe called again. This is so hard for him. I hope it gets better for all of us.

E mail from my niece, Stacey:

My Precious Aunt Deane,

I know this must be very hard for you. I cannot even begin to imagine your pain. I have seen firsthand how effective trained professionals can be while caring for Alzheimer's patients. I am relieved that you are able to get physical rest, as well as mental rest.

I know you miss Uncle Joe, but you have missed him for a very long time. Please know that you have done the right thing for both of you. My heart aches with you.

You are strong, Aunt Deane. I am like you and proud to be so. I wish I could dry your tears, but I know they will continue for some time. I hate that you're in such pain, and I hate that Uncle Joe has Alzheimer's, but your decision is best for you both.

I love you and Uncle Joe.

Love Always,
Stacey

May 17, 2010—Monday

The sun is out, the humidity is very high, and I am falling apart. I know taking Joe to his new home is the right thing for me, even though my heart feels as if I have broken it. I wonder if it is the right thing for Joe. I ask myself, "Do I, as a loving wife, put myself first, knowing it probably won't be comforting to the love of my life?" I am lost. I am alone with feelings of despair and a sadness I could never have imagined. The pain and tears are washing over me like a flood. I am drowning with every sob. I have no words to express the pain, this anguish of a broken heart. I sit here and try to find the words to tell the world how I'm feeling, what I'm feeling, and I don't think there is a word in any dictionary that could describe the pain of this grief.

Joe is still alive, but lives in another house. He will be cared for there. It isn't that I don't want to care for Joe, but I knew a week ago that if I continued, I would be sick. Our children don't need both of us sick and in need. Joe has Alzheimer's, but he is lucid a good part of the day. This is what makes this separation so sad. I know he is wondering where I am. Joe tells me all the time that we are lovers, and I belong to him. I do belong to him, and Joe is mine, all mine, lucid or lost.

I had to direct him to brush his teeth and help him get dressed. I had to be patient, because he had slowed down to a snail's pace. I fed him, talked to him, and had to be with him all the time unless our help was here. Even with help, Joe would call for me. When he went to bed, I had to go to bed to appease him. Joe would get up to go to the bathroom, but he didn't know where the bathroom was. If I got up, he would wake up and, being the caring, loving gentleman he is, he'd ask if I wanted him to go with me to make sure I didn't fall. I probably haven't slept all night for several years. I didn't realize I was this tired until after Joe moved to the Alz Care residence.

I called the church to tell them where Joe was now living. Ann and Steven Davey came out to be with me for over an hour. Our kids called to ask about me. Mindy spent the night with me. How am I doing? Not good at all.

Joe called Mindy, wanting to know where she was. This isn't going to be a piece of cake. I cannot stop crying. I don't want to bring Joe home. I know I can't take care of him. I was close to hitting a concrete wall if I continued having Joe at home with me. I am tired. I am lost. I am so very, very sad. My marriage as it has been is forever gone. How do I find peace and comfort living apart from my Joe?

May 19, 2010—Wednesday

I went to visit Joe today. It was so good to see him. He doesn't understand why we don't sleep in the same bed anymore. That makes me sad. Unless I spend the night with Joe, we will never sleep together again. The visit went smoothly, which surprised me, and I didn't cry when I left. After this move, I must find some joy every day in my life. Sad as it is with Joe gone, I have many years of loving memories to help me see the joy.

May 20, 2010—Thursday

I visited Joe again. I go because I want to see him. Jody and I took him to Cotton Patch for dinner. Joe asked where I had been, and he wanted to leave with me when Jody and I left. I departed with a heavy heart. We will go see Joe again tomorrow.

May 21, 2010—Friday

When Jody and I went to see Joe today, Joe told us he was in San Antonio, and that he was in the Army. He wanted to show us around town. We stayed for an hour or so, and then went home and rested. We picked Joe up around 6p.m., and met Mindy and Jim at Casa. Joe told Jody he had hurt his back while skating in the Ice Capades. Joe said the guy skating in back of him told Joe to turn a flip if he wanted to win. So Joe said he turned a flip and hurt his back when he fell. For the Alzheimer's patient, maybe sun-downing isn't all bad and depressing. Maybe sometimes it's even fun because they live in a fantasy world.

May 23, 2010—Sunday

I didn't visit Joe today. Without him around, my world is stagnating. I went to dinner with the Burleson's. I stayed up and watched a movie until 1a.m.—something I haven't done in years.

May 25, 2010—Tuesday

I visited with Joe yesterday. It is always hard for me to leave him. He doesn't understand why we don't live together anymore. I am exhausted, and can't stop crying. Mindy and Jim visited Joe at Alz Care today.

May 26, 2010—Wednesday

I visited Joe today. He talked about sex a lot, but that is not unusual for him. He again asked why we sleep apart, and asked me if our marriage was over. The sleeping together is over, but my marriage to Joe will never be over. The union will continue into Heaven.

May 29, 2010—Saturday

I went to the twins' high school graduation last night. Joe would have loved going.

Tonight, the Burleson's picked me up, and then we picked up Joe. We had a great dinner at the Olive Garden. Ed and Carolyne went inside Alz Care to visit with Joe, and when we left, Joe wanted to leave with us. It hurt me so much. I don't want him to think I don't want to be with him. I do want to be with Joe, but I can't be his 24/7 caregiver anymore.

May 31, 2010—Monday (Labor Day)

I sat in Joe's chair all day, thinking about and remembering all the wonderful times we've shared through the years. Memories keep the head from a tail spin.

June 2, 2010—Wednesday

I had a very good visit with Joe today. I think he may be adapting to his new home. I am not even close to adapting to the separation, even though I know it is best for him and better for me physically and mentally. The pain I feel every waking hour will probably not go away until the final curtain is closed. So, I will try to make the best of it and be thankful I can still be with him and love him. While I was at Alz Care, Mindy came by to visit Joe.

June 3, 2010—Thursday

Every day I am tired and want to sit, cry, or nap. I am lonely. Joe doesn't know where I am. We are both unhappy. I ask myself why I moved Joe away. I know why—because I had come to the end of my rope. But I hate being apart from Joe.

June 4, 2010—Friday

An e mail to Dicque:

I am not handling this separation from Joe very well. I didn't know what a broken heart felt like until now. I cry, I weep, I cry out loud. I scream, I am not happy, I must get through this.

I have had some really good visits with Joe. I want to crawl in bed with him again. Joe asked me how I know where he is. He looks good, but he always has. I am not close to finding any kind of peace or joy. I didn't know grief was this disruptive. It sweeps over me, and I can't control my tears. I may be okay one minute, and then I turn into a grief-stricken woman the next second. I am so tired. My doctor told me I was overwhelmed with the move, the change, and the years of dealing with Alzheimer's. My assignment is to look for a silver lining under this heavy blue cloud.

Love You,
Deane

E mail reply from Dicque:

As good as it can be sometimes, Life is cruel. Love is cruel. I wonder why Love is part of the human condition. Is it a trick of Nature just to get us to breed and replenish the Earth?

Yours and Joe's love for each other has endured for so many years only to end up like this—together, but apart. I can't imagine your sadness, unless I try to put myself in your place for a minute. Even that attempt for me is too terrifying.

I think of you ever so often throughout the day, but my prayers don't reach that far up to help.

Love Forever,
Dicque

E-mail from Kathy (we met her and her husband, Gary, on the Italy tour):

Oh Deane,

This is the hardest part of life—to lose your soul mate in mind, but not body. I think that, because you had such a wonderful and enriching life together, it makes it that much tougher. You were lucky to have more than most couples have in a lifetime. I am so sorry. The strength, love, and support from your family and friends are what you need to help you deal with this.

My heart aches for you and Joe. Please know that I am always thinking of you with love.

xoxo,
Kathy

June 5, 2010—Saturday

Ed and Carolyne picked me up this evening, and we picked up Joe to have dinner at Casa. Joe thought he had been playing in a band. He thought I should know where the band job was last night. Joe thinks about music jobs a lot. He wonders if the band has anything booked. We took him back, and, as usual, he didn't understand why he couldn't come home with me. My heart aches for both of us.

I have to see this through. I must always look at the moments. Joe seems to be settling into his new home away from home. When Joe looks at me and tells me he doesn't understand why we aren't living together, I want to scream that I don't understand why either. Why us?! Why you?! Why me?! My heart breaks like a glass that has been stepped on and crushed into a thousand pieces. My heart aches for all we've had. My heart is being broken every time I leave Joe and walk back into this life alone. A life we have shared for almost fifty-nine years. We still love just as we did in the beginning. We are apart in body, but always together in spirit. I am so sad. This doesn't make sense to me. If Joe wants to be with me and I want to be with him, I ask myself why I moved him away from me. I know why—because my body couldn't continue on the same path I have been on for the past seven years. I finally faced reality that if I continued taking care of Joe, I was going to crumble into a thousand pieces. I think it would be hard for Joe if I couldn't visit him, love him, and let him know daily how much he means to me. I would die a slow death if I was unable to see him several times a week to reassure him, as well as myself, that our kind of love will ease our pain.

I need something to ease this pain of grief. I need my Joe, but this miserable disease has forced me to make this heart-wrenching decision for us to live apart. I ask God to hold my hand until the end of our journey.

June 6, 2010—Sunday

Here I am, another day of sitting. I took a nap. I went to dinner with the Burleson's. I did not go see Joe. I called and was told he roamed most of last night.

June 8, 2010—Tuesday

Today, Mindy and I picked up Joe to run errands. Mindy explained to Joe that Dr. Morledge gave her and Dena orders to move him to his new home because I needed rest. She told him I wasn't happy either, but in order to give us more years on this earth, this arrangement was made by her and Dena.

June 11, 2010—Friday

I dread going to see Joe, but I want to see him. Today, I stayed for three hours. The visit was good. Joe had an accident. While he was showering, I left. When he got out of the shower and missed me, he called me. He was angry, saying ugly things and wanting a divorce. In the future, should I slip out, or should I tell him I'm leaving? If I tell him I'm leaving, he will ask to go with me and ask why we don't sleep in the same bed anymore. Either approach can be good or bad. We are both affected by living apart.

June 12, 2010—Saturday

The Burlesons picked me up this evening, and we picked up Joe for dinner. I stayed with Joe for a little while when we took him back to his new home. Mindy then picked me up at 9p.m. We left, and Joe was fine when we left him this time.

June 13, 2010—Sunday

The girls at Alz Care called me, because Joe was trying to break out a window to leave. Jackson and Eric were visiting me when I received the call. We all went over to Alz Care together. After a short time, I figured out Joe was upset with me because he thought he was at his office and I had no reason to be there. I left, and the boys stayed. I think Joe calmed down a short time after the boys left.

June 15, 2010—Tuesday

When I got in bed tonight, I had a meltdown. Any time I go see Joe, I am weary of leaving, knowing the departure will be hurtful for him. But if I don't visit Joe, I am sad. Either way, I am stressed. I am hanging by a thread.

June 14, 2010—Wednesday

Mindy and I took Joe out to dinner tonight. When we took him back, I had to explain again why I was leaving and why he slept at the retirement home. When I finished my explanation, he looked at me and said, "I guess I drew the black bean."

June 19, 2010—Saturday

Jody and I took Joe out to dinner tonight. When we took him back to Alz Care, I had to explain again why he is living at the retirement home. He said, "I guess I lost again." That statement, along with the black bean comment, didn't make me feel good. It made me wonder if Joe thinks I have given him the short end of the stick. I know in his earlier mindset he would have told me to find him a place to live separate from me, but Joe hasn't been that logical in at least six years. I wonder every day how I will end up, mentally, while living apart from Joe. We may live separately, but we will never be separated in our hearts and spirits.

June 20, 2010—Sunday

Today is Father's Day, so the girls went over to visit with Joe. They stayed a couple of hours. At one point, Joe asked where I was. He thinks about me, and I think about him minute to minute. We are both sad. I cannot be his caregiver any more. I wish our visits didn't end with his questions of why he can't come home with me.

When the girls left, Joe asked Amanda, a girl who works there, why they had to leave. She said they had to go feed their husbands. Joe said, "I wish I were their husbands."

June 22, 2010—Tuesday

Joe called Mindy tonight, and he was vulgar and mean over the phone. Does this happen more often when he is out with us, or does it happen when he can't see us? I don't want to stop seeing him, but I don't want to make it hard for him and us when we do see him.

June 23, 2010—Wednesday

Thoughts I discussed with my grief counselor:
1. Should I try to re-create the feeling of our home when I am at the Alz Care home with Joe?
2. By trying to do it all, have it all, and give my all to Joe, am I setting a pace that leaves us both scattered and exhausted?
3. My life has shifted. How do I welcome the change, and shift along with it?
4. I realized this morning while thinking of Joe that I visit him more for his own good than for mine. If we have a good visit, and I can leave without him making me feel that I am keeping him locked away from me, then it is a welcoming visit.
5. If the visit has gone well, but my leaving concerns him with many questions, this visit sets me back.
6. Everyday my first and last thoughts are of Joe. I think of him throughout the entire day. When Joe sees me, his face lights up. I kiss him and cuddle with him, and these are natural feelings I love and need from him. But all the time we are together, he asks why we are apart. This isn't good for me and probably not good for him. Thirty minutes after I leave, he forgets I've been with him, but sometimes it takes me 24 hours to recover.
7. I want and need to hold him and comfort him, but how do I get the good part and brush off the toxins of the visit?

8. My love for Joe is constant and never changes.

9. Facing the fact that our marriage as we've known it is over and that we will never live at the same address is truly hard to bear.

10. Every time I visit Joe, I know I have to let go of what once was, but hang on to the good parts that remain. But even voluntary letting go is not without sorrow and many tears.

11. Why? How? How long? Am I up to the challenge I am facing? These are the questions I constantly ask. My heart still isn't in the decision I've made for Joe, but my newfound health gives me the courage to follow through with my choice. It still doesn't take away any of the pain.

June 26, 2010—Saturday

I visited Joe from 1p.m. until 6p.m. today. When I got there, he was sleeping. I woke him up, and he asked if I was his daughter. I told him I was his wife. I curled up beside him in the chair. He patted and stroked me, and said it felt like old times. Joe napped some more, and I curled up on the bed. He kept opening his eyes to see if I was still there, then he'd go back to sleep. I stayed to have dinner with him, and he introduced me to everyone as his sister. Today was the first time since he has moved that he didn't know me. When I got home, I sat in his chair until bed time.

June 27, 2010—Sunday

I had a meltdown today. The reality of this journey is much too vivid and painful. Every time I leave Joe, it is a mini death, and sadness sets in. If we had buried Joe, there would have been the certainty of an end. But he is living, breathing, and he needs to see me. I need to see him too, even though it hurts. It is amusing how people expect me to shake off my grief and get on with my life after only six weeks of living apart from Joe.

June 27, 2010—Sunday

Dear Dr. Morledge,

Moving Joe to his new Alz Care residence was and is the most heart wrenching decision I have ever had to make. It has been six weeks and four days since Joe left our home. It is no easier today than it was the day he left. I know I can't be his caregiver and retain my physical and mental health. If I don't go see him, I am sad. When I do see him, I am sad.

The grief which follows a natural death eventually diminishes with time. When I visit Joe and leave, I experience a mini-death, and the sadness renews itself each time. I remind myself to look for the joy and the love that Joe and I share. I know that joy is waiting to be discovered even in the sadness of the moment.

I urge all couples to talk, reminisce, and not miss a day of loving and caring for one another.

Knowing you gives me courage.

> *Lovingly,*
> *Deane Johnson*

June 28, 2010—Monday

I face another day away from Joe. I washed, swept the patio, and watched TV.

Sunday was a long, long day. I watched four movies. For me, this isn't giving in to my grief. It is enjoyable. I haven't been able to watch a movie from start to finish in several years.

I cooked fish and green beans for my dinner. I miss Joe more when I cook. Tonight I had a strong need to call Joe. He has a wonderful sexy voice. The reality of never having a phone conversation with him again is what started my melt down. I worry that if I phone him, his reaction may be negative, asking me why we have to live apart. Then it could cause him to sun-down. So I cried, felt sorry for us both, and made it to bed for a night of sleep.

June 29, 2010—Tuesday

Today Dr. Morledge asked me when I was going to publish my journal. I told him sometime soon. I informed him that I had no idea I was as tired and exhausted as I have been. He told me I needed a lot more rest.

June 30, 2010–Wednesday (The Final Entry)

I am grateful for my doctors, my children, and my friends who have encouraged me to keep resting. No one can know the stress I have lived with these past years. I spent this afternoon with Joe. I enjoyed being with him, sitting close, and being patted. It would be more pleasant for both of us if Joe could enjoy the moment and stop asking questions like, "When are we going home?" and "What are we doing tonight?"

We watched TV, and, as usual, our conversation was very limited. Joe asked why he is living here, and where I live now. He worries about his car. He asked where our children are. Joe does not remember he has fourteen grandchildren unless I bring up their names. He never knows who the grandchildren's parents are.

It is always the same when I leave. Joe wants to go with me. But twenty minutes after I leave, Joe probably has no memory of me visiting. The emptiness fills me, but I try to leave that feeling at the door and not bring it home with me.

I'm sure if any of us were put in Joe's shoes, we would ask all these same questions. Imagine being at a residence and not knowing how you got there. You don't recognize anyone, and you don't know where your spouse sleeps. You don't know how to go home or even if you'll ever go back there again. Writing this sounds as if the person with Alzheimer's is living a nightmare. Here is what I think: I can't dwell on Joe's questions. I know Joe doesn't think in a logical way. I don't mean he isn't smart. He is a loving, intelligent man, but he has Alzheimer's. This is the only way I can cope. I tell myself that once Joe asks a question, he quickly forgets what the question was. Then a few minutes later, he asks the same question again. If Joe wonders if he will ever go back to his home, by the time he finishes the question and I explain the whys and wherefores, Joe looks at me and says he doesn't understand my explanation. For me to keep my sadness and stress to a minimum, I have to remind myself that Joe has Alzheimer's. Yes, Joe forgets. And even though I remember the heart-tugging questions, I know Joe will leave the Alzheimer's zone and in the next minute or two he will be content.

Mindy and Jim are leaving for Colorado for eight days. I want all my children to carry on with their lives. I don't want our needs to take them away from their children. Sure, I miss them, but I have missed each of them since they left for college, so this is nothing new.

This will be the last day I write in this journal. In my next journal, I will attempt to put in words the daily trials of Joe and me living apart, and how I look for new joys each day.

Journaling has been therapeutic for me, and it has shown me the valleys and peaks of Alzheimer's. I can look back and see how I've faced my days and how I've found a way to enjoy simple moments. Living apart is another hurdle we face. I will no longer feel Joe's hand on my back when we sleep or feel his foot searching for mine in the middle of the night. I visit him often. He still knows me and responds to our whistle. We find comfort sitting together, quietly, shoulder to shoulder, maybe holding hands and exchanging a kiss. We both find joy just being side by side. Each page of this journal reminds me of the love Joe and I share and that our love will burn forevermore. Robert Browning said it best:

Grow old along with me; the best is yet to be,
The last of life for which the first was made.

The last of life is precious, even with Alzheimer's.

Reflections From Joe's And Deane's Children

Jody's Reflection

Hundreds of people were in attendance for the retirement party, a happy occasion marking the end of the working part of Dad's life and the beginning of the unknown—retirement. Dad had always been petrified of retirement. He was like many of his generation that thought people retired and, soon after, died.

During the celebration of his years as a practicing attorney, Justice of the Peace, and District Judge, Dad was introducing one of my sons to several of his friends. "One of the best football players in the history of Odessa Permian," he proudly proclaimed. Dad had never been to Odessa, much less to an Odessa Permian High School football game. We had never lived in Odessa, and my son had never played football for the school. That was the first time I thought there may be a problem.

Within months, Dad was at a neurologist's office, not sure of the town he was in, the day of the week, the month, and unable to draw a clock. Alzheimer's was a new member of our family.

How did our family accept the disease? There was an ample dose of denial. For some, denial lasted years with the constant thought that Dad was just forgetting in a normal way and the neurologist had "made a mistake." Dad was immediately placed on a cocktail of medications. The medications, his love for music, and Mom's constant attention allowed him to function at a moderate level for several years. Mom was the caregiver. My sisters live close and were a huge help, but in the end Mom provided care every day. She would have it no other way. My brother, sisters, and I watched as Dad's mental abilities slipped, and Mom's frustration grew. It became obvious that Dad needed more care than Mom could provide, and that Mom was deteriorating as the caregiver faster than Dad was with his brain disease. One second, Mom was at the end of her rope and ready for Dad to move, and the next she was overwhelmed by guilt and the feeling that she was letting her life partner down.

We kids had multiple meetings and discussions. We recognized what was happening, and our initial thought was to take control and force the issue of Dad moving to an A-facility. Had there been any significant danger to Mom or Dad, we would have intervened, but until that significant danger existed, this was Mom's decision to make. We watched, supported, talked, visited, and continued to let Mom know that moving Dad out of their home was totally her decision. In hindsight this was a very important decision, and the right one for our family. Ultimately, Mom was able to make the decision herself, and Dad was moved to an Alzheimers' home.

Dad's pride and joy was his intellect and his musical talents. He was the first in his family to graduate from college, become a lawyer, a judge, and a world class musician. Alzheimer's robbed him of his intellectual skills, but did not rob him of who he was, his love of music, and his sense of humor. To this day, he stops in his tracks if he hears a trumpet blasting a high note, and can laugh with the best of them when something tickles his fancy.

Everyone faces hardships. We are not defined by the hardships we face, but by the manner in which we respond to the hardship. Despite the tragedy of the disease, there have been positives that have resulted from this journey. Our family recognizes that life is precious and we should accept each day as it is presented to us. Our family was able to allow Mom to make the key moving decision in her own way in her own time which allowed her to move from the guilt phase to the grieving phase. Since Dad's diagnosis, I have had a real and compassionate relationship with him that we, frankly, didn't have before. There is a spiritual aspect to our relationship that was probably always there, but only recognizable in the last few years. When I visit him, we can sit in silence. It is not uncomfortable. In fact, it is just right. He may not know my name all the time, but he truly knows who I am. There is a connection that is not about words or deeds; it is just about being, and being with people that you love. Dad and the A-disease have taught me to be in the moment and not spend every waking minute fretting the past or fearing the future. The A–disease forces the moment, and it is a good lesson.

Today, Dad lives in an Alzheimer's facility. We visit him regularly. He is physically healthy, he is content, he is well cared for, and he is still Dad, whether he knows your name or not.

-Jody (Joe Jr.)

Barry's Reflection

When my father was diagnosed with Alzheimer's, I, like other members of my family, was in denial as to the severity of the disease and whether or not he really had it. Like most family members with an early diagnosis of Alzheimer's, I was relieved that he did not have a terminal disease commonly associated with physical pain, like Lou Gherig's disease, pancreatic cancer, paralysis, or many other physically painful terminal illnesses.

As it turned out, I would rather have had a diagnosis of any other disease than this cruel and unpredictable mental illness. I had some experience with mental illness because two of my law partners had family members with mental illness. They had told me that mental illness affects the entire family, that the whole family would become somewhat mentally ill. I just did not think Alzheimer's (hereinafter Alz) fell into the category of mental illness that my law partners' family members suffered from—e.g., schizophrenia, paranoia, bi-polar, etc. However, as time went by, I realized Alz is actually just as bad as any mental illness and has the same effect on the family as the other mental illnesses mentioned above. Like all mental illnesses, they are so unpredictable in that the sick loved one may seem fine one day and digress horribly by the next time you see them. This gives the family member so much false hope only to be sorely disappointed the next time you see your sick family member. This is the way I was with Dad. At times, he seemed so normal, and I would hope against hope that maybe the Doctor was wrong about the diagnosis, and then the next time I would see him, I would usually get a painful dose of reality—the reality that he had a terminal illness that was going to gradually eat his brain away and cause his death around 10 years from the date of diagnosis, which was in December, 2003.

In the early stages of his disease, I did enjoy talking with him about old times after his short term memory was gone. His long-term memory stayed in tact much longer, and ironically, it seemed he actually remembered more details about events and people's names from 40 years ago than he remembered before he got sick. He told some really funny stories about his life that I had never heard before. When I realized his long term memory was still functional, I tried to talk about times long ago, in his childhood or adolescence. It was amazing what he could remember from way in the past, and with his wonderful sense of humor, it was fun to hear the stories. Of course, this insidious disease ultimately took his long-term memory as well.

I was extremely worried about my mother trying to take care of him, as I had always heard that the caregiver usually dies first. We tried to encourage her to get help with a support group or other methods, but she chose to wait until the later stages so that she would not go against my Dad's strong desire for nobody in Waco to know he had Alz. Mother was afraid if she went to a support group, it would uncover his secret. My father was a very prideful man and did not want anybody to know he had Alz. I did not agree with this and thought we should tell his close friends and elicit as much help from friends and others as possible, but it was not my decision to make. I honored Mother's and Father's wishes, but believe in retrospect this put way too much pressure on Mother and kept her from getting the help and support she needed to assist her through many lonely and difficult years as his main caretaker.

As time went by and he became worse and worse, it was as though he died every day. My mother went to a funeral every day, and my sisters, who lived in Waco, went to that same funeral most every day. I was having other issues in Dallas that kept me from helping as much as I should have. I lost my job and went through a divorce, which either prevented me from helping as much as I needed to, or provided an excuse for me not to have to face the emotional trauma the disease was putting on my mother and sisters. I had and still have a great deal of guilt about this.

A visit home before he got sick was always a fun and joyous occasion. I now dreaded going to their house. The pain of watching my father slowly waste away, with his personality changing dramatically at every visit, and my mother doing the best she could to care for him was extremely difficult to watch. After four or five years, it was as though he was dead. The man we all knew was gone, but there was no way to put a punctuation mark on it and mourn his death.

The mourning and grief of losing him continued in our family and still continues on a regular basis. It finally got to the point last year (2010) that my mother gave her permission to put him in a nursing home. In retrospect, this decision was probably a year or two too late, but better late than never. Her life has hopefully somewhat improved in that she now has some time to herself and a sanctuary away from the hell of the disease. I was finally able to have a conversation with my mother after Dad went to the nursing home.

I always derived a great deal of comfort in having my father just 100 miles away, whether we saw each other often or not. We had a good relationship and good friendship. He was the funniest man I have ever known. He was a great comedian and had a wonderful sense of humor. He was always fun to talk to, and he was so knowledgeable about Law and Life in general. It was great to be able to call him with a question or just discuss some problem with him. We would both usually laugh really hard, though he sometimes was ready to get off the phone fairly quickly, especially if he was watching his beloved TV. He used to say he loved TV so much that he wished he could get inside it.

He was great fun to watch TV with—football games, golf, or anything. He would often narrate the shows, or have something to say about whoever might be on the tube. He even enjoyed commercials.

It is extremely difficult, even as a 55-year old man, to accept the reality that he is gone. It is like this black hole that can never be filled. I am grateful for the time I had with him, but realize life will never be the same.

-Barry

Mindy's Letter

The daddy/daughter bond is a strong one. I have always admired and been proud of my Dad. He has forever been my protector and my hero.

Late one night in July of 2008, my Dad broke my heart. My Mom had gone to bed (recovering from brain surgery), and my Dad and I were watching TV. He began to make inappropriate advances toward me. I tried over and over again to convince him I was Mindy, his daughter, his third child. In his mind, I had become his girlfriend. I began to panic. This man, my Dad, who has always been an authority figure in my life became (in my mind) a predator. I was scared and repulsed. My mother heard my panicked voice and came to my rescue. I became hysterical and called my husband to come spend the night at my parents' house and protect me. The next day, by myself in my backyard, I had a private funeral for my Dad. He was gone.

That was the first time in my life that my Dad didn't know me. My Dad would never have treated me that way. I became angry and depressed. I did not want to be alone with my Dad. I was scared of him. That man looked like my Dad and sounded like my Dad, but *my* Dad was not there. Even though I've watched this disease slowly take over my Dad these past seven years, nothing prepared me for the shock of that evening and the trauma it caused in my mind.

Then, one day I woke up and realized this situation was not about me. My Dad is a human being with a monstrous disease. I was ashamed for blaming my Dad for something he had no control over. He would be horrified if he knew what had happened. I now look at his memory loss as both a tragedy and a blessing. The tragedy is that he doesn't know his family anymore and doesn't remember events in his life. The blessing is that he doesn't suffer from guilt or embarrassment regarding his hallucinations and paranoia. He isn't burdened by sadness from realizations of what he's missing. When I spend time with my Dad now, I try to make him feel normal, important, dignified, and loved. We laugh a lot. I like to sit and hold his hand.

There is a permanent sad place in my mind to which I cannot let myself go very often. I've learned to block out the painful part of this journey. I take comfort in knowing that my Dad seems very happy and content with his life. He lives in a wonderful Alzheimer's home where he is constantly nurtured. My Dad still has his famous sense of humor and impeccable manners. He still plays his trumpet and remembers all of his big band tunes. I love my Dad deeply, and am grateful for the moments I still have with him. I will always be a "daddy's girl," and he will always and forever be my hero.

-Mindy

Jim Wren's Letter (Son-In-Law)

For me, Joe has always been "The Judge." I've known him for years longer than I've known my wife. As I went through law school, he was already a lawyer and Justice Of The Peace of long standing, extremely well known and highly respected in the Waco legal community. He was funny, fair, and there was no arguing about either point.

As luck would have it, I was the defense attorney in the first jury trial in his court after he won election as the district court judge. And from the first, there was no question how his court would be run. Lawyers, litigants, and jurors would be treated with respect. He set the tone in that regard, and he absolutely expected all others in his court to exhibit that same professionalism. Whether lawyers agreed or disagreed with his rulings, absolutely no one questioned the personal integrity and desire for fairness behind his rulings.

Later, after I began dating and became engaged to his daughter, he made it clear that he would no longer be presiding over cases in which I was involved. Yet for me he was still The Judge. As our relationship deepened and evolved over the next decades, I was able to see how some cases affected him, particularly cases involving children. He wanted—desperately at times—to get those cases right, and I could see the gut-twisting anguish when he felt that the justice system couldn't fix the problems that ran much deeper in people's lives.

Even after his retirement from the bench, and even as Alzheimer's has taken its toll, he has remained The Judge. I've never referred to him, in or out of his presence, by any other name. It is a name of respect and of endearment. It says not just who he was, but who he is. There is no claim of perfection. What exists is a man who desires in his deepest soul to get it right, and to ease the pain with some humor in the process. My first word each time I see him is "Judge!" As all else slips away, he knows who he is. It's hard to watch a lifetime of memories and learning leave. But at his essence, the integrity and fairness and honest heart for people that have laid hold of him for a lifetime still come through. To the last, he is reminding me that the core of a man is the last to go.

-Jim

Dena's Letter

I remember after my dad retired, my mom would talk about how daddy could not remember little things like where the pens were kept, where the paper was, and how to look up a phone number. We all just assumed it was because he had always had people doing things for him. When he was at work and needed to make a call, his secretary would find the number, dial it, and pass it through to him. Okay, well, if we are being honest, my true thoughts were, "He is a man and doesn't pay attention. People are at his beck and call waiting on him. Men are not multi-taskers. He is just used to being waited on." Period.

Unfortunately, that was not the case. I also remember on the day he retired from being a District Judge, the county commissioners honored him for all his years of service. We all gathered for the event, and I was really nervous for him because I could sense something was not right. He was going to have to stand up in front of everyone and speak, and I thought, *How is he going to do this?* He was obviously nervous and slightly confused. As well as I can remember, I think he made a nice speech. But I remember it being awkward and really, really sad. My dad was walking away from forty years at the court house as Justice Of The Peace and District Judge. It was time for him to retire and begin a new season of life. Little did we know that this new season of life would suck.

Thinking back, I cannot help but wonder what emotions daddy was going through in his own head when he first started experiencing the Alzheimer's symptoms. I am confident he was way too prideful to admit he was having any confusion or memory problems. I wonder how many times he wanted to say, "You know, I got confused driving to work this morning" or "I couldn't remember where to turn." I have talked to several attorney friends of mine who have said, "Now that we know he had the beginning stage of Alzheimer's, things which were happening in the court room now make sense." It makes me sad to think of how scared and alone he must have felt having all the Alzheimer's symptoms and not being able to tell anyone, "I am scared. I don't know what is going on." He must have felt so alone. My dad was King Of The Castle, had a lot of pride, and to admit something was wrong was just not something he would do. Sad, isn't it? And the ironic part of it is that my mom would have been the first to take care of him, coddle him, nurture him, tell him everything was going to be okay. It would have eliminated a lot of frustration on her part. She is thinking, "Can this man pay attention at all? Geez, he has selective hearing." I just wish we had all clued in sooner. Even when you see obvious symptoms, you cannot help but go into complete denial. Because things like this only happen to "other people."

So I cannot think of just one worst part of this crappy disease. There are SO many. One of them was picking him up from his home, knowing it was the last time he would ever be there, essentially tricking him into leaving, all the while knowing my sister and I were taking him to live in an Alzheimer's home. I have never seen my mother cry like that. Gut wrenching. Pain unlike anything I have ever seen. I watched part of her die that day, but I knew this was the only way she would truly live again. Being his caretaker was slowly stealing her own life. We (adult children) had to sit back and wait for his leaving to be her idea. That was the only way it would ever work. And it was hard to watch.

Finally, Mom reached her breaking point. We had it all planned out. It was time. We were all in agreement that this was the absolute best thing to do. We had watched my mother take complete care of him for far too long. She was exhausted, and we were exhausted just watching it. I was sad for her to lose Daddy, but excited for her to regain part of her life back.

So, how did the day go? It stunk. On every level, it was awful. My sister and I had decorated Daddy's new room to make it feel homey. We drove through Sonic to get him a diet coke and told him we were going to visit one of his old musician friends. There we were, sitting in his new room, we showed him his new comfy chair, with his room decorated with music and family pictures. Ready for this? He had a moment of lucidity. He was figuring things out. Wow, this was crappy timing. We told him that mom was really tired and that this was where he was going to stay for a few days until she felt better. Mindy and I were not at all prepared for him to put 2 and 2 together. Oh, but he did. He said he felt tricked, that he had drawn the bad card, that we were trying to get rid of him. Oh my goodness, now what do we do? We tried to explain, but the bottom line is, there was nothing we could say to make it better. We had to leave him there. We had to walk away, and leave him in that room. The girls that work there said he sat in that chair most of the day waiting on my mom to come pick him up. However, we all knew this was the next step, and it was past time. He adjusted fairly quickly.

Here we are almost one year later. He's doing great at AlzCare. How am I handling it? I am not in denial about his disease, I just don't like to see it. I know, I know, who does, right? I do not go see him very often. I average a couple of times a month, or less. I don't want to see him like this. It is too hard. He may know me, he may not. You never know who you are going to get: the sweet and tender daddy, the angry daddy, or the "judge" daddy?

One time I went to visit, and he thought I was the local prostitute. He used horrible, vulgar language, told me in detail what I was going to do with men that were waiting for me. I tried to get him on another subject, but he was determined that I was a hooker. Now, I know that is not my dad. I know it is Alzheimer's. I am in no way offended. It is just that the man who took me to Johnson's Ranch every month to ride horses when I was little is not there anymore. He is long gone, and that is hard for me to accept. When I go see him, I see a man that looks like my dad, but it's not *really* him. I just wish we could go back and say the things to each other that needed to be said. Like, "I love you." I never said it. The few times I said it to him, he teared up and could not speak. So, I know it was in him, it was just hard to say. I wish I could have him back.

I have never cried about my daddy having Alzheimer's. I have definitely been sad, but would never allow the tears to flow, until today. I miss him.

-Dena

A Story About Joe And Me

I celebrated my 81st birthday this year. I realize that there are some landmarks in my life, things that stand for the memories where life has been so full. One of those is the house I still live in, the house that my husband Joe and I scraped money together to build for our family in the 1960's. And as you step into the front door of our house, there's a large, life-sized, black and white portrait framed on the wall to the left.

The picture shows a smoky night club scene from more than sixty years ago. There's a very young and very handsome young man playing the trumpet. A band member sits at the piano a little further behind, with a bass player to the other side, and a guitarist. I've been in love with and married to that trumpet player, Joe Johnson, for sixty years now.

Since this book is, at its core, a love story, let me tell you the story of The Picture (*see P. 13 to view the photo).

In the spring of 1950, I was 19 years old. My daddy had died when I was nine after years in and out of hospitals from being gassed in the trenches in World War I. My mother and I would have been called homeless today, but in those days we simply moved from home to home of various family members, surviving, until my mother remarried. And it was lonely. There weren't any brothers or sisters to move with me.

But I loved to dance. Wherever we lived, my mother made sure I attended dance class.

I got the chance to attend Baylor University after high school. I loved all the activity in the dorms, classes were okay, but most of all I looked forward to my drama classes and dancing lessons. A date to go dancing was the best.

Casa Blanca was a night club across town from Baylor, sitting on a hill above Lake Waco. In the spring of 1950 I was lucky enough to have my date take me to Casa Blanca. When we walked in the door, a trumpet solo filled the air. By the time we made it through the crowd to the dance floor near the stage, the band leader was singing "A Cottage for Sale." He was handsome, impeccably dressed, with the trumpet tucked under his arm. I danced, hoping to make eye contact with the trumpet player. It didn't happen. I had no idea who he was when we went in, but I knew his name when we left.

Joe was only two years older than me, but he had already spent time touring as a professional musician. Later I discovered that he had grown up in Waco, in a family that also struggled to pay the bills while his father's health failed. Although music was not a family priority, his parents had purchased a coronet for one of Joe's older brothers, hoping that it would help the brother overcome asthma. Joe's brother showed no interest in the coronet, but Joe did. He taught himself to play. Before high school, Joe was playing everything he heard or could hum. He started playing trumpet professionally at age fourteen and would continue playing professionally until the age of eighty-one.

After high school, Joe started touring with the Art Mooney Band out of New Orleans, and then joined the Sonny Dunham band in New York. But after traveling with the bands for eighteen months, rarely seeing daylight, he came back home, organized the Joe Johnson Orchestra, began playing every weekend at Casa Blanca, and enrolled in Baylor University to major in music. He didn't stay in music school long (classical training seemed a little dry for a jazz band trumpet player), and he decided to go to x-ray school. Weekends stayed the same, however. He was at Casa Blanca and soon, as a result, so was I.

After that first spring night, if a date wanted to take me dancing at Casa Blanca, my answer was yes. One night, my date called Joe Johnson to our table and introduced us. I was star struck. I wanted to make a good impression, and, instead, I sat there smiling and speechless.

Joe didn't know where I lived, didn't know my phone number, and it was obvious he didn't ask.

That didn't keep me from dreaming. I became a regular at Casa Blanca. I flirted, smiled, tried to make eye contact with Joe, and hoped. On December 31, 1950, the moment seemed to arrive. Joe motioned for me to come to the band stand, and he asked if he could kiss me Happy New Year. It was only a moment, but it was our first kiss.

And then he didn't call.

By the end of January, I figured that he was not going to call me. That's when I decided to take The Picture. I did something I had never done before. I hired a photographer to take pictures of the band and of Joe. Maybe Joe would never call, but at least I would have a picture of him.

It's funny how one thing leads to another. After the picture, Joe did call. He didn't have a car. The few dates we had were double dates with friends. If we didn't have plans with friends in the evenings, we sat outside in lawn chairs to talk and steal a kiss. There was no air conditioning in those days, but the Texas heat was no deterrent for us. We were falling in love.

War was exploding in Korea. Joe received his draft notice and reported to Fort Sam Houston in San Antonio, which was several hours away by bus. When he could, Joe would come home on Friday afternoon late and leave to go back on Sunday evening. In July of that year, Joe proposed. The summer heat permeated the house, but I didn't feel the heat, only Joe sitting close to me. He didn't get on one knee. He simply sat beside me, asked me to marry him, and my yes was immediate.

We had no money, the Korean conflict made our future uncertain, and Joe's mother wanted us to wait until Joe was discharged in two years. I wanted to get married the next day.

I wasn't worried about money, but Joe was. Joe and I discussed marriage all of July and into August. He struggled with the decision about timing. One Sunday afternoon before Joe left to go back to Fort Sam Houston, Joe's older brother Roy and his wife asked me to come in the back yard with them. We sat on the grass in the shade of a back yard cottage. Roy's advice to me was to get a job out of town. Roy said that if Joe couldn't see me every weekend, Joe would make the right decision for us. I knew what I had to do.

I caught a bus to Dallas on Monday, and asked the taxi driver to take me where I could apply for an airline hostess job. I was quite naive to think I could get a job that day. In the August heat I walked from one end of Lemon Avenue to the other, applying for a job with every airline there. My last stop was Pioneer Airlines. Luck was on my side. I was hired to start to work in a week.

On the bus from Dallas back home to Waco, I sat by a lady who told me she had a room for rent in Dallas. We agreed on the price, and she gave me a key and the address to my new home. I caught a bus back to Dallas the next day with my clothes, and after buying my uniform I was a working girl. I trained on the job.

September and October were lonely months away from Joe. I wondered if I had done the right thing. What if he was shipped to Korea and something happened to him? We wrote letters and had several weekend phone conversations. On October 20, 1951, Joe called and asked, "Do you want to get married next Saturday night?" He knew my answer would be "Yes-yes-yes." I wired my boss that I quit my job, borrowed a dress, called our preacher, ordered flowers and a cake, and Joe and I were married at my home October 27, 1951. We had a one night honeymoon with a five dollar room at the Falls Hotel in Marlin, Texas. We paid fifty cents extra to rent a radio for the night. Joe went back to Fort Sam Houston on Sunday.

Joe shipped out for France in May 1952, assigned as an x-ray technician. The morning he left was a sad, hard day. I went back home, got a job, and lived with Joe's family. We wrote to each other every night, counting the days until Joe got his discharge. Then on my birthday in August, Joe wrote saying he had made arrangements for me to join him in France and asked me if I'd be willing to come over there. I, of course, was thrilled.

Joe was waiting for me when I stepped off the plane in Paris. Our hotel was not fancy, but I certainly didn't care. The hotel did have an elevator, a community bath down the hall, occasional heat, a feather bed, and a continental breakfast every morning. My dream had come true.

Joe and I spent our days at sidewalk cafés sipping cokes. Imagine our shock to learn a coke in Paris cost seventy-five cents! We strolled up and down the Left Bank looking at art, went to museums and the top of the Eiffel Tower, watched children sail their boats in the large fountains, and enjoyed every minute being together again. This was a honeymoon of honeymoons.

Joe had rented a duplex for the winter in the summer resort town of Fouras, France. We lived a few blocks from the ocean. We walked the beach when the weather permitted, we explored the quaint city of Fouras, and we enjoyed this adventure far from Texas. Our duplex had electricity, and cold, running water was furnished. We also had a roll away bed, feather mattress, three chairs, a table, a two burner hot plate fueled with propane, no refrigerator, no hot water, coal burning stove in the kitchen that we never learned to use, and a stove in our main room without a working flue. For entertainment, Joe played his trumpet and I guessed the tune. From time to time, Joe would play as a featured performer with a local French jazz band. Being in France with Joe was as if we had a fence built around us separating us from the world.

Joe's orders to return to the U.S. came in May of 1953. Our fence was coming down, and we were moving back to reality.

We docked in New York City after eleven days on a ship. Joe had lived in New York when he played with the big bands of Art Mooney and Sonny Dunham. For eight days, he showed me the city and introduced me to its music. To our surprise, Stan Kenton and the Four Freshmen were playing at Bird Land. Joe and I spent five evenings at Bird Land. The admission was $2.50 a person.

We came home, Joe started back to college, organized the Joe Johnson Orchestra, and learned I was pregnant. Joe (Jody) was born in 1953, and Barry in 1956. Joe finished college in 1956 and went to work as a TV reporter. Our daughter, Mindy, was born in 1957. Joe worked full time at KWTX, and booked the Joe Johnson Orchestra every weekend, but we needed more money to take care of our family of five. Joe was offered a job as news reporter at the Waco Tribune Herald for an additional five dollars a week more than his current salary. He went to work covering the court house. After a few years, a local judge began to encourage Joe to go to law school. In 1962, Joe decided to take the risk. He applied for law school and simultaneously decided to run for election as Justice Of The Peace. Joe borrowed five hundred dollars to buy cards and emery boards for us to hand out, enlisted friends to help, and we plunged into the campaign. He won the race by a two-to-one margin while he was starting law school. At the same time, I found out I was pregnant with our fourth baby. In January of 1963, Joe began his job as Justice Of The Peace, his band played three or four nights a week to provide income, and Joe was attending law school. Our baby girl, Dena, was born in 1963.

Joe received his law degree from Baylor in 1964, and practiced law for the next twenty-two years. We built our home shortly after Joe finished law school, where The Picture now hangs inside the front door.

Joe made friends easily. People loved him. He was funny, he was intelligent, and he was fair with people and treated everyone the same. And his music was first rate.

He was elected Judge of the 170th District Court in 1986. He served there for sixteen years. As Joe neared retirement in 2002, we dreamed big dreams of the next stage of our life together.

Then we found out Joe had Alzheimer's.

-Deane Johnson

If you would like to invite Deane to speak at your event, please e-mail her at: *deane@deaneandjoe.com*

Visit Deane's website at:
www.deaneandjoe.com

Made in the USA
San Bernardino, CA
08 January 2014